Understanding Dementia

Alan Jacques
MB BCh DPM MRCPsych
Consultant Psychiatrist, Royal Victoria Hospital, Edinburgh

Churchill Livingstone

EDINBURGH LONDON MELBOURNE AND NEW YORK 1988

CHURCHILL LIVINGSTONE
Medical Division of Longman Group UK Limited

Distributed in the United States of America by
Churchill Livingstone Inc., 1560 Broadway, New York,
N.Y. 10036, and by associated companies, branches
and representatives throughout the world.

© Longman Group UK Limited 1988

First published 1988

ISBN 0-443-03586-5

British Library Cataloguing in Publication Data
Jacques, Alan
  Understanding dementia.
  1. Dementia
  I. Title
  616.89   RC524

Library of Congress Cataloging in Publication Data
Jacques, Alan.
  Understanding dementia.
  Bibliography: p.
  Includes index.
  1. Dementia. I. Title. [DNLM: 1. Dementia.
WM 220 Jl9u]
RC521.J33 1988   616.89   87-11807

Produced by Longman Singapore Publishers (Pte) Ltd.
Printed in Singapore

Preface

This book aims to help the increasing body of professional and other workers who come into regular contact with dementia sufferers and their carers in the course of their work. It is not a practical manual, but a guide to understanding. It is not a textbook for any individual professional group, who will have their own language, and their own procedures, but is an attempt to give a common understanding to different professions and agencies who work together in solving the problems of dementia.

I have taken a problem-orientated approach to the assessment of dementia sufferers and recommend this as a good basis for effective management (Table 9.7). Although none of the management techniques discussed will lead to a cure for the common causes of dementia, it is nevertheless possible to be optimistic about some degree of improvement in many cases.

Some of the views expressed here are personal, but much of the book is based on the expertise of my medical, nursing, occupational therapy, psychology and social work colleagues at the Royal Victoria Hospital, Edinburgh, the contribution of primary care teams, social workers and home care staff of the North of Edinburgh, and the daily experience of numerous sufferers and carers. I acknowledge with thanks my continuing education by all these people, and the continuing influence of Sam Robinson who set the standard for psychogeriatric care in Scotland.

My special thanks are due to Moira Burke and Margaret MacDougall, who have enthusiastically and tirelessly helped in the preparation of the text.

Throughout the text I have referred to dementia sufferers as female. This is not in any way sexist. It is simply a reflection of the fact that the great majority of sufferers *are* women. I have also tended to call them patients rather than clients. This is not only because I am a doctor, but is justified because dementia is an illness which can cause great distress to sufferers and their carers.

I hope that the ideas which I put forward here will have some influence in increasing awareness of and interest in dementia, and will encourage a positive approach to the problems of its sufferers as individuals.

Edinburgh 1988

A. J.

Contents

1

What is dementia?

Dementia is a syndrome which may be caused by a number of illnesses. The main features are of a progressive decline in all aspects of cerebral function

There are still many people who think that dementia is a normal part of the ageing process. Many assume that any psychological change or eccentricity in old age is evidence of dementia and therefore untreatable. This sort of 'just old age' generalization should now be out of date. For we are able to define the syndrome of dementia reasonably well both by saying what it is and by saying what it is not, even if there is some woolliness at the boundary.

In this chapter we shall look at what dementia is and the illnesses which cause it, by examining the definition above more closely. In the past few years some real progress has been made in understanding its commonest causes. This is a developing area of research, which may eventually lead to effective treatments for a group of disorders which are becoming increasingly common as more people survive into extreme old age.

DEFINING DEMENTIA

Dementia is a syndrome

Firstly, what is the evidence that dementia should be seen in terms of illness and disease at all? It is, after all, quite a common condition and could be seen as a variant of old age, at the end of a spectrum of normality, rather like extreme shortness of stature or very high intelligence.

Using the word 'illness' implies that a patient's condition is out of the ordinary, not part of her normal life, and that there are some detrimental effects — the symptoms and signs or *clinical features* of the illness. A *syndrome* is a characteristic pattern of symptoms and signs which can be caused by one or other of a number of illnesses. Each of the illnesses should have a clear underlying pathology, whether that be organic or psychological, and we should be able to explain how that pathology leads to the clinical features of the syndrome.

An abnormal condition

Dementia is not a part of normal life. Indeed, it is important to note that at all ages, even into the 80s (or the 100s for that matter) dementia is a minority condition (Table 1.1). The figures quoted are taken from a community survey of elderly people in Newcastle-upon-Tyne. They show that the vast majority of elderly people are *not* deteriorating mentally.

It is not therefore justified to say 'when I am old and demented' as if the one condition followed the other inevit-

Table 1.1 Prevalence of dementia in the community (adapted from Kay D W K et al 1970 Comprehensive Psychiatry 11:26)

Age group	Percentage of the group who suffer dementia
65–74	2.5
75–79	8
80 and over	18
Over 65	6

These estimates include mainly severe and moderate cases; many mild cases are not included as diagnosis is unreliable at this stage.

ably. Nevertheless dementia *is* quite rare in people under 60 and it increases in prevalence at later ages — the older one is the greater the *risk* of suffering dementia. So it is an illness of old age but not a normal part of it. The difficulty in definition only comes when we try to draw a clear dividing line between what is normal in old age and what is dementia. We will discuss this more fully in Chapter 2.

Detrimental effects

Throughout the book I will be emphasizing the detrimental effects of dementia on its sufferers and those around them. No-one can doubt the magnitude and importance of these effects; they constitute an enormous challenge to health and social services and to the population as a whole.

In terms of seeing dementia as illness, however, the most significant effect of all is its final outcome — it kills the patient. It was shown about 30 years ago that dementia markedly shortens expectation of life (Table 1.2). Those patients, who were in long-stay psychiatric wards, were mostly in their 60s and 70s. When this study was repeated in the hospitals of the late 1970s where the average age had risen to over 80 this shortening of life was less apparent. Perhaps better hospital conditions contributed, but it also may be that dementia beginning in a person who is in her 80s is a less killing disease (see p. 22). This thought should make us pause when we consider that there are now very many more people in this older age group (Table 3.1), and that many of them have few available relatives to support them.

Table 1.2 Life expectancy of dementia sufferers

Group studied	Average expectation of life (years of remaining life)	
General population at birth	Women 77 yr	Men 72 yr
General population at 65	Women 16 yr	Men 12 yr
Dementia sufferers in the 1950s (mostly in their 60s and 70s)	2–5 yr	
Dementia sufferers in the 1970s (mostly in their 70s and 80s)	5–10 yr	

A pattern

The main purpose of this book is to show the characteristic pattern of symptoms and signs in dementia. The word 'dementia', implying loss of the mind or loss of mental powers, describes the basic process well. Other terms which have been used such as *chronic brain syndrome* or *chronic cerebral failure* are no better and no worse.

Although I will emphasize how complex the mental decline is in a particular individual, there are clear common features in all patients.

These are due to progressive damage to widespread areas of the brain, and are different in pattern and degree from the normal changes of old age. Attempts to divide up dementia by identifying sub- types such as apathetic dementia or paranoid dementia have been partly successful, but there is no evidence that any of these sub-types is more likely to be caused by one particular underlying disease.

Whatever the cause of the dementia, the basic pattern of symptoms and signs and the pattern of decline are roughly the same; in other words, it is a syndrome.

Causal illnesses

The second part of this chapter will describe a number of illnesses which can cause the syndrome of dementia. Some of these illnesses have other characteristic symptoms in addition to those of dementia, but in all of them the typical overall decline in cerebral function occurs. We will see that each of these illnesses has a characteristic pathology which can explain that decline.

So, there are some good reasons for thinking of dementia as illness — its minority occurrence, its detrimental effects, its causes and their characteristic pathologies. Thinking this way has stimulated research and encouraged attempts at treatment. It has helped make dementia respectable.

Dementia is a progressive decline

From normal to death

Before the dementing process began, the victim was, of

course, her normal self, and this 'normal' is the baseline from which we measure how much she has changed. At the end of the illness the patient is dying. What actually causes death in simple dementia is not clear. Presumably, as more and more functions decline, the brain's ability to adjust to changes in the environment (for example, by heat regulation or control of the heart or breathing) eventually deteriorates to such an extent that life can no longer be supported. These final stages leave the patient bereft of mental powers, unable to understand, communicate or reason, needing everything done for her, incontinent and chairbound.

But between the normal self and this terminal vegetable-like existence lie several years of very gradual deterioration. She is dement*ing*, not dement*ed*, and we should try to emphasize the gradually progressive nature of dementia by using the former term.

Presenting complaints

Within the basic syndrome of dementia there is considerable variation in the rate of the decline from person to person, and in a particular individual the different brain functions may fail at different rates. This is obvious even at the beginning of the process, for there is a variety of ways in which dementia declares itself — the presenting symptoms (Table 1.3).

Most people are aware that memory loss is an important feature of the illness, and this is, indeed, often the first complaint. But, in looking back, relatives may recall other more subtle changes in personality, personal habits or moti-

Table 1.3 The presenting symptoms and signs of dementia

Losses	Memory impairment
	Decline in self-care
	Decline in management of one's affairs
	Decline in work performance
Change in behaviour	Uncharacteristic behaviour
	Social withdrawal
	Personality change
	Mood change
	Paranoid ideas
Acute confusion which fails to clear	Due to illness
	Due to a change of environment

vation, which perhaps started several months before the decline in memory. Sometimes it is an uncharacteristic way of behaving (e.g. hoarding, wandering, shoplifting, disinhibited behaviour) that shows that something is wrong, sometimes it is an episode of more acute confusion.

But unfortunately, early referral for assessment and help, or referral when the decline is steadily and quietly progressing are not usual. For in many cases the insidious onset, the common attitude that it is 'just old age' and the assumption that nothing can be done conspire to keep relatives from complaining. The patient herself may not be aware of the changes, may try to cover them up out of embarrassment or may share her relatives' unhelpful attitudes, so that she does not complain either.

Crises

Furthermore the gradual decline in the commonest form of dementia — Alzheimer-type — does not usually bring any very dramatic or sudden changes during its course. The result is that action is demanded only when there is a crisis (Table 1.4). Indeed, the dementia may only be very belatedly recognized when one of these crises occurs. In multi-infarct dementia, the second commonest cause of dementia, the patient's state may suddenly take a turn for the worse because of a small stroke, and so medical crises are more common.

Table 1.4 Crises in dementia

Crises of behaviour	Gas left on
	Water taps left on
	Lost in the street
	Disinhibited behaviour
	Shoplifting
Crises of care	Death of carer
	Illness of carer.
	Relative arrives on holiday
	Relative goes on holiday
	Home help goes
Medical crises	Drug mistake or overdose
	Physical illness
	Acute confusion due to physical illness
	Strokes in Multi-infarct dementia

However, the usual crises of dementia are about quite extraneous events, as Table 1.4 shows; and not only are they of different origins but they demand action from different agencies. In the crises of behaviour it may be the police, the housing department or social work department who are called; in crises of care it is the social workers or primary health care team; in crises of health the primary care team or hospital. To make matters worse a health problem is sometimes referred to social work, a crisis of care to the police, and so on.

Management of the decline

Of course, crises cannot be totally avoided. But one of the vital tasks facing the professions and voluntary organizations who deal with dementia is to shift the focus away from crisis management on to management of the slow decline; for it is this decline which *is* dementia and which causes the main burden of care, 24 hours a day, 7 days a week for several years. This shift will be achieved when we persuade relatives to make that early referral, when proper assessment is seen as a worthwhile effort by general practitioners and other professionals, and when this assessment takes into account the multifactorial problems of dementia, needing multidisciplinary solutions.

When a crisis does occur, it should be seen not necessarily as a reason to rush an old lady into long-term care, but rather as a reason for a cool review, by all involved acting together, of those multiple problems and of the care being given. Surprisingly often, the crisis can be survived and better care organized for the future.

Ribot's law

This cooler look at the problems facing a patient whose entire brain is failing requires some understanding of the course of the illness. A generalization called Ribot's law is helpful, though only as a generalization. This law states that functions of the brain which develop later in life are the first to deteriorate when widespread damage occurs.

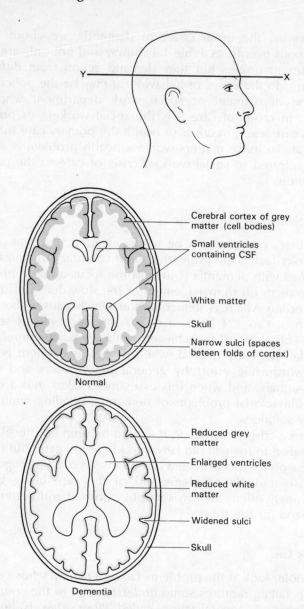

Cerebral cortex of grey matter (cell bodies)

Small ventricles containing CSF

White matter

Skull

Narrow sulci (spaces beteen folds of cortex)

Normal

Reduced grey matter

Enlarged ventricles

Reduced white matter

Widened sulci

Skull

Dementia

Fig. 1.1 A horizontal section through the brain of a normal person, and a similar section through the brain of a sufferer from severe dementia. CT scan and NMR scan pictures are similar to these and can provide evidence of dementia.

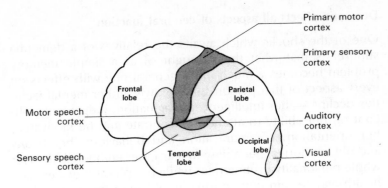

Fig. 1.2 The surface of the cerebral hemisphere from the side, showing some specific functional areas.

When we look at the most specific and localized functions of the brain, for example hearing or sight, which have very direct and definable representations in small areas of the cerebral cortex (Fig. 1.2), we find them unaffected at least in the early stages of most dementia, as Ribot's law suggests. So, the damage of dementia tends to affect the co-ordinating and connecting functions of the brain more than these specialized areas which are fully developed very early in life. Ribot's law also suggests that, as a rule, we would expect that urinary incontinence would begin to be a problem at a later stage than decline in memory, and that faecal incontinence would develop later than urinary incontinence. If this general sequence is not followed, and the patient is, say, incontinent at an early stage of dementia, or incontinent of faeces while still continent of urine, then we should think again.

Despite Ribot's law, there is actually a lot of variability in the course of dementia. So when a symptom does not fit the usual pattern of decline we may merely be seeing that variability. But it could be that there is a quite separate diagnosis as well as the dementia; the early incontinence could be due to a urinary tract infection, the early faecal incontinence due to constipation, for example. The other diagnosis is in danger of being missed if we think that anything that looks like part of dementia *must* be dementia without trying to fit it into the overall pattern.

Dementia affects all aspects of cerebral function

One of the shocks which awaits the relatives of a dementia sufferer is that what they thought of as a simple memory problem becomes a much more general one with effects on every aspect of that person's life. Slowly all her mental faculties decline — her intelligence, imagination, judgement, self-control, her ability to attend, concentrate and be motivated, her orientation, communication and behaviour, her habits and old memories, her ability to learn, her emotional life. Her whole personality disintegrates while her physical powers and health may remain quite normal until late in the illness. Relatives need to be warned early about these changes so that they can be prepared and know how to look for help.

From the professional's point of view there is also a problem. It is relatively easy to test certain brain functions — intelligence, memory, constructional skill, and test them reliably. It is rather more difficult to measure behavioural changes. It is almost impossible to measure judgement or imagination. We are in danger of concentrating in dementia on the measurable, useful though the tests are, and forget the more subtle general changes.

In fact, to understand the basic process of dementia, we need simply to think of all that the upper parts of our brains do, as that is the list of functions which are likely to decline. It is the whole personality, all that was ever learned, the basic controlling and organizing functions of the cerebrum which are affected. We will detail these changes in Chapters 4 and 5.

General damage and patchy damage

We will see however that, as research clarifies the illnesses of dementia and their effects, we need to clarify the words 'all aspects' of cerebral function. For Alzheimer-type dementia does not damage every bit of the cerebral cortex equally (p. 16) and there is even more patchy, though widespread, damage in multi-infarct dementia (p. 26).

Nevertheless, when we look at the more general functions, such as intelligence, thinking and understanding, what has been called the 'law of mass action' seems to apply in dementia. This states that <u>when there is widespread damage</u>

to the cerebrum there is proportionate damage to these general functions. So a lot of little injuries, even if they are patchy, act as if they were one general injury.

CAUSES OF DEMENTIA

If we see dementia as a gradual decline in the function of the cerebrum, then to understand its causes we must look for causes of gradually increasing cerebral damage (Table 1.5).

Pre-senile and senile dementia

In the past, the syndrome of dementia was sub-divided into a pre-senile and a senile type, with the dividing line drawn at an age of onset somewhere around 65 (Table 1.6). There is no doubt that this division into sub-syndromes had some value; the frequency of the various causes of dementia differs between the two age groups, and there are different effects on the family and social life of a person of working age and an elderly retired person. However, as a consequence of the sub-division, younger, pre-senile patients may have been referred more often to neurologists, while the older, senile patients were seen as suffering from the ordinary problems of old age and referred, if at all, to one or other of a wide variety of agencies, to find the solution to the crisis of the moment. The result has been a clearer definition of the dementia syndrome in younger patients with an emphasis on its more neurological manifestations and some vagueness in describing 'senile dementia'.

There are now good reasons for questioning the pre-senile/senile sub-division. In the first instance, when examined closely, the pattern of symptoms and decline is actually very similar in patients who develop dementia in their 50s and those who develop it in their 70s, even if the social effects are different. Attempts to distinguish the genetics of the two conditions have brought confusing results but the case for a 65 break is, at the least, unproven. Most crucial is the fact that it has been impossible to distinguish any major differences between the pathological changes in the brains of the two groups.

Table 1.5 Causes of dementia

	Type of damage	Illness	At least partially reversible at present	Treatment
Common	Plaques, tangles and transmitter defects	Alzheimer type dementia (ATD)	–	–
	Multiple infarcts	Multi-infarct dementia (MID)	–	–
Uncommon	Transmitter defect	Parkinson's disease	+	(Antiparkinsonian drugs do not help the dementia.)
	Physical damage	Normal pressure hydrocephalus	+	Shunt operation
		Repeated head injury	+	Stop boxing
		Slow growing brain tumour	+	Operation
	Toxic damage	Aluminium poisoning (dialysis)	+	Stop dialysis
		Wilson's disease	+	Penicillamine
		Alcoholism	+	Stop drinking
	Genetic disorder	Huntington's chorea	–	–
		Wilson's disease	+	Penicillamine
	Infections	General paralysis of the insane	+	Antibiotic
		Creutzfeldt-Jakob disease	–	–
	Nutritional deficiency	Vitamin deficiencies	+	Vitamins
	Endocrine disorder	Hypothyroidism	+	Thyroxine
		Parathyroid disorder	+	Medical or surgical treatment
	White matter damage	Multiple sclerosis	–	–
		Binswanger's disease	–	–

'Senile'

The distinction between pre-senile and senile dementia was further muddled by the use of the term 'senile dementia' to describe an *illness* which is the most common cause of senile dementia the *syndrome* (Table 1.6). It is thus unclear, when a person is described as suffering from senile dementia, whether it is merely being stated that they are over 65 and dementing (the syndrome), or whether they are suffering from the specific disease which we now call senile dementia of Alzheimer type (or, less clumsily, Alzheimer-type dementia).

The word 'senile' has in any case been much misused in common speech, sometimes vaguely and sometimes pejoratively. It can mean old, more likely to happen in older people, physically decrepit, mentally infirm, or just plain unwanted. In the absence of clarity we would be better to avoid its use altogether. We will drop the pre-senile/senile distinction, look at dementia as a whole and examine the underlying diseases.

At all ages the commonest causes are Alzheimer-type dementia and Multi-infarct dementia. We will first describe these conditions and then look at the relatively uncommon causes.

Alzheimer-type dementia (ATD)

When Alois Alzheimer first described this illness in 1907, the population structure and pattern of mental illness were very different from today. In Britain and other similar countries the proportion of the population aged over 65 was around 5% (today the figure is over 15%), and the proportion over 75 was very much smaller; so small indeed that it was not even measured in the census, a statistical anomaly whose present day importance was only fully recognized in the mid-1970s (Table 3.1).

In asylums 80 years ago, inmates included two important groups who would have been described as 'demented'. Firstly, there were sufferers from chronic schizophrenia, or dementia praecox — the dementia of adolescence. The decline in drive and emotion, and the typical social withdrawal of the schizophrenic were seen as a form of dementia. However, pathologists failed to show any significant damage

Table 1.6 Old and new terms in dementia

Terms for the syndrome	Sub-syndrome	Causal illnesses	New term for illness
Dementia Chronic brain syndrome or Chronic cerebral failure	Pre-senile dementia	Alzheimer's disease	Alzheimer-type dementia (ATD)
		Arteriosclerotic dementia	Multi-infarct dementia (MID)
		Other causes in **Table 1.5**	
	Senile dementia	Senile dementia	Alzheimer-type dementia (ATD) *or* senile dementia of Alzheimer type (SDAT)
		Arteriosclerotic dementia	Multi-infarct dementia
		Other causes in **Table 1.5**	

in the brains of schizophrenics at post-mortem and the changes began to be seen as purely functional, not structural. It is interesting that in the last few years the debate has reopened, with some claiming that there is, after all, brain damage of some sort in chronic schizophrenia.

The second group, possibly up to one-third of the inmates, would be suffering from a true dementia, but not Alzheimer's disease. This was the dementia of tertiary syphilis — general paralysis of the insane (GPI — see p. 32). One of the most important episodes in the transformation of psychiatry from a humanitarian custody of the insane to a medical speciality was the linking of GPI to infection with syphilis, the finding of the bacterium which causes syphilis in the brains of GPI patients and the subsequent beginnings of effective treatment for a previously incurable illness.

Alzheimer, then, was picking out from among these dementia sufferers another smaller group of patients who were suffering profound dementia not due to syphilis and with different pathological changes. He was describing pre-senile patients, but it was early seen that many senile dementia cases were largely indistinguishable from his pre-senile cases. It was only with the development of specialized neurochemical tests and electron microscopy in the last two decades, leading to more detailed pathological studies that the identity of the two conditions was confirmed.

In Alzheimer's day there would anyway have been few senile cases in the asylums. The relative rarity of very old people and the existence of large numbers of potentially supporting relatives, coupled with few expectations of treatment, kept sufferers in their own homes with their own families.

Pathology

We are now able to define the pathology of Alzheimer's dementia quite clearly, although the distinction from normal ageing at the early stages remains a problem.

Shrinkage. The cerebral hemispheres are shrunken and lose weight (Fig. 1.1). This change is more easily definable in younger sufferers and in them can be easily displayed by brain scanning using computerized tomography (CT scanning). However in older patients and in normal, undemented, old people there is more variability in brain size and demonstrating the shrinkage of ATD is less reliable.

Site of the damage. The cause of the shrinkage lies mainly in the cerebral cortex, the grey matter coating the cerebrum which contains many millions of nerve cells or neurones; though the white matter, which consists entirely of nerve fibres, or axons, is also shrunken. It is still not absolutely clear to what extent it is the death of nerve cells, or their shrinkage, or changes around the cells which cause the general shrinking of cerebral grey matter in ATD, for measuring the number of cells in the cortex is difficult.

A variety of studies show that in ATD, damage is concentrated in certain areas of the brain, especially the temporal lobes, which include the hippocampal region, an area specifically involved in recent memory function, the frontal lobes and, to a lesser extent, the parietal lobes (Fig. 1.2). In these areas cell deaths have been demonstrated. We will see how this pattern of damage is reflected in the main clinical features of dementia in Chapters 4 and 5.

Plaques and tangles. More significant than the actual death of cells may be the widespread evidence that neurones, and especially their endings and connections, are degenerating. The characteristic pathological finding under the microscope in Alzheimer's dementia is of *argentophil* or *'senile' plaques* and *neurofibrillary tangles*.

The plaques are of obscure origin; they show up with silver stains under the microscope (as the name argentophil suggests) and contain degenerating nerve endings and a variety of the substance amyloid which is often found in connection with inflammatory changes or degeneration. The number of plaques is greatest in the areas of brain where there is most shrinkage and the number of plaques is proportional to the degree of intellectual decline in a dementia sufferer. Plaques are also present in small numbers in the brains of undemented old people.

The tangles also relate in numbers and site to the damage of dementia. Normal old people only develop tangles in the hippocampus. It is still not absolutely clear of what the tangles are composed, but one likely possibility is that they are the remains of damaged parts of neurones, for they lie within the cells.

The existence of plaques and tangles implies that there is a reduction in the number and variety of nerve cell connections throughout the areas that are damaged.

Neurotransmitter deficits

Further important evidence comes from the chemical study of the neurotransmitter substances which convey the signal that there has been a electrical change in one neurone to another (Fig. 1.3). In the brain there are a number of these transmitter substances and each cell transmits one specific transmitter chemical. The transmitter causes an electrical change in a second neurone, making it either more or less likely to release *its* chemical transmitter. The entire functioning of the brain depends on millions of these messages between neurones.

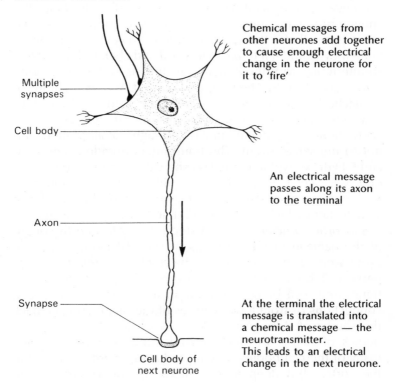

Chemical messages from other neurones add together to cause enough electrical change in the neurone for it to 'fire'

Multiple synapses

Cell body

An electrical message passes along its axon to the terminal

Axon

Synapse

Cell body of next neurone

At the terminal the electrical message is translated into a chemical message — the neurotransmitter. This leads to an electrical change in the next neurone.

Fig. 1.3 A schematic diagram of a typical neurone.

Acetylcholine. The enzymes which are involved in the creation of transmitters and their breakdown show whether a particular sort of nerve cell in working or not. It was shown about 10 years ago that the enzymes related to the neuro-transmitter acetylcholine (ACh) were greatly reduced in the brains of ATD sufferers, particularly in the most affected areas such as the hippocampus.

It was already known that drugs which interfere with acetyl-choline can cause confusion as a side-effect or in overdose, ('anti-cholinergic' substances include many anti-depressants and some anti-Parkinsonian drugs). There has also been evidence that substances which stimulate or simulate the action of acetylcholine in the brain (cholinergic substances) may actually improve memory temporarily in non-demented people. There is even an old wives' tale that fish, which is rich in choline, the precursor of acetylcholine, is 'brain food'.

It began to look as if ATD was a specific disorder of acetyl-choline-producing nerve cells and their connections. We could guess that if the acetylcholine nerve cells die or degenerate they would fail to pass electrical and chemical messages, so interfering with the general functioning of the cerebrum.

Multiple deficits. This simple theory of ATD as a failure of acetylcholine nerve cells has had to be modified by further research. This has shown that other transmitters as well as acetylcholine are affected in ATD, though not all of them and not to the same extent. The transmitters noradrenaline (NA) and 5-hydroxytryptamine (5-HT) show decline in a similar sort of way to acetylcholine; the transmitter gamma-aminobutyric acid (GABA) also declines somewhat; and the substance somatostatin which is probably a transmitter is reduced.

Subcortical nuclei. The next step is to try to find the origin of the damage to these groups of cerebral nerve cells. The axons which end is synapses in the cerebral cortex come from nerve cell bodies within the cortex, making short connec-tions, from cell bodies far away in the cortex, making long connections or from lower centres of the brain. To trace back the source of damage in ATD we need to look for the cell bodies of Ach-, NA- and 5-HT-releasing neurones. In fact, many of the cell bodies of Ach-producing neurones lie not in the cortex, but deep in the middle of the cerebral hemi-spheres, in a small nucleus of cell bodies called the nucleus

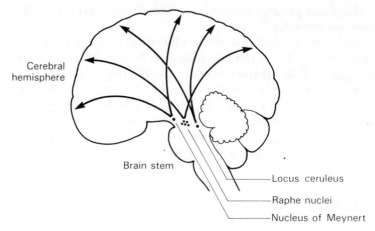

Fig. 1.4 Cell bodies in subcortical nuclei have long axons which end at synapses in widespread areas of the cerebral cortex, the areas which are affected in Alzheimer-type dementia.

basalis of Meynert. Here there is obvious death of neurones in ATD cases. The same goes for other nuclei in the centre of the brain for two other affected transmitters — the locus caeruleus for NA, the raphe nuclei for 5-HT (Fig. 1.4).

Possible causes of ATD

So, ATD, which originally was seen merely as a shrinkage of the brain, is now seen as a disorder of a few types of neurone. It may be a disorder of particular cells in subcortical nuclei, resulting in a failure of transmission at the ends of their axons, at synapses widespread throughout the cortex, resulting in the pathological changes in the cortex and the consequent decline in cerebral function. It may be that the basic damage is to the nerve endings where the plaques and tangles are. Whatever the site, we now need to look for what is causing the damage to these particular types of neurones. A number of possibilities have been considered.

Genetic factors. There are a few families in which there seems to be a strong hereditary factor, passing on ATD from generation to generation. However, looking at the majority of ATD sufferers in the population, there are problems in working out genetic influences, even though ATD is such a common disorder.

Firstly, the boundaries of the illness are difficult to define; secondly, absolutely definite diagnosis before death is not yet possible; thirdly, since dementia usually occurs later in life, many potential sufferers die of quite unconnected illnesses before they would develop the dementia, and it is impossible as yet to know whether these people carry the genes of ATD or not.

On balance, it is thought that there is some genetic contribution to ATD, but its nature is still debated. Some say that a first degree relative of an ATD sufferer (that is a child, brother or sister) is four times as likely to develop the illness as someone without an affected relative; others that the likelihood is doubled. Whatever its degree, the effect of this genetic factor is presumably either that more damage occurs to the groups of nerve cells which degenerate in ATD, or that those cells are more susceptible to damage.

Chemical damage. A variety of poisons from outside the body, especially metals such as lead or aluminium, are known to damage nerve cells, and it could be that one or other of these poisons builds up in the neurones in ATD. A type of dementia found in the Pacific island of Guam is possibly due to metal poisoning from the local water.

There has been considerable interest in aluminium since it was found to cause brain damage when it got into the bloodstream of renal dialysis patients. And there is some evidence of increased aluminium in the senile plaques of ATD sufferers. It may be that this is due to taking in too much aluminium in the diet, but it is more likely to be due to a failure to get rid of normal amounts of aluminimum from the brain (as for copper in Wilson's disease, p. 30).

It is also known that older neurones build up presumably from internal sources, more complicated, possibly toxic chemicals which cannot be disposed of. These include the substance called lipofuscin commonly found in the neurones of older people. Some of these substances might be damaging to the nerve cells.

Infection. A cell may also be damaged by the invasion of viruses which interfere with its normal workings. Many viruses can damage brain cells either directly in encephalitis or more indirectly by some sort of allergic reaction. The discovery that the rare Creutzfeldt-Jakob type of dementia is caused by a very slow acting virus, or something like a virus, called a 'prion', led to a hunt for viruses in ATD cases. So far no virus has been identified but the virus theory is still a strong possibility.

Chromosome damage. One common idea as to how any of these three types of factor could impair the function of a nerve cell is by damage to its central directing mechanism, the DNA of the chromosomes. This is the genetic material which determines which proteins a cell produces, when and in what amounts, to maintain the cell's structure and function.

A genetic cause would imply some increased susceptibility of the chromosome material to damage or disordered function. A chemical or infective agent might directly damage the chromosomes. Encouraging this idea of abnormality of the chromosomes in ATD is the surprising finding that all sufferers from Down's syndrome (mongolism), which is caused by a clearly definable chromosome abnormality, if they reach their 40s, develop in their brains the typical pathological changes of ATD, and almost identical neurotransmitter losses as well. The typical chromosome abnormality of mongolism in not, of course, found in ATD cases.

Treatment of ATD

Research into the causes of ATD has expanded very rapidly in the past few years. There are 3 reasons: first, the rapid increase in the number of dementing people because of population changes; second, the growing feeling that dementia should be looked on as an illness, not just old age; third, the chemical findings which led researchers to believe that an effective treatment might now be found.

When it was first shown that acetylcholine action in the brain was impaired in ATD cases, the exciting possibility emerged that a treatment might be found which could replace the deficit and stimulate the acetylcholine neurones into action. The discovery that L-dopa could do this for the neurotransmitter dopamine in Parkinson's disease provided a hopeful model. However, so far, clinical trials with the precursor of Ach, choline, and with related substances have brought only a few hopeful results.

There are good pharmacological reasons why choline might not be effective and, of course, the deficits in 5-HT, NA and somatostatin must complicate matters. Even if we could find ways to replace lost transmitter action, however, we would only be reducing the *effects* of the nerve cell damage, not stopping that damage. We would therefore expect such treatment to give temporary relief and simply to delay the decline. But the benefits for the large number of sufferers from this long-lasting disease would surely be worth the effort. The effects on our attitudes to old age and 'senility' bear some thinking about. Clearly initial hopes have had to be modified as the pathology has become clearer and more complicated, but it is most important that this basic research progresses while the task of coping with the effects of dementia continues to be the more urgent priority.

'Young-old' and 'old-old' Alzheimer-type dementia

Before leaving the subject of ATD it is worth noting a further direction in which research is heading. Although the distinction between senile and pre-senile ATD now seems pointless, a dividing line at a greater age is emerging (Table 1.7).

This later division was first suggested by the term 'benign senescence', used to describe 'old-old' people who, in their 80s and 90s, begin to develop a less profound memory disorder than younger ATD sufferers, with less widespread

Table 1.7 A comparison of 'young-old' and 'old-old' ATD

	Younger patients (onset below 75 yr)	Older patients (onset above 75 yr)
Life expectancy	Shortened	Less shortened or normal
Damage to cerebral cortex cells	More widespread More severe	More localized Less severe
Neurotransmitter losses	More transmitters affected	Mainly acetylcholine
	More widespread damage	More like normal age changes

effects on general brain function, and who surprisingly have a more normal lifespan than younger patients. It was next suggested that those younger patients, with an age of onset mostly in the 60s, tended to suffer more damage to their parietal lobes (see Fig. 1.1). This suggestion has been at least partly confirmed by CT scanning and the pathological changes.

The neurotransmitter evidence 'adds further support — in older ATD patients, with dementia starting in the 80s and 90s, the transmitter loss is less widespread over the brain and is more confined to the acetylcholine neurones. In fact, this old-age ATD bears a much closer resemblance to changes in the brains of normal older people of the same age, who usually have some degree of acetylcholine loss, than does the multiple transmitter loss in younger patients.

So it may be that we should divide Alzheimer-type dementia into two varieties: a more malignant, early or 'young-old' dementia and a more benign, 'old-old' dementia. The implications of this for health and social services are enormous. Not only is dementia a commoner problem among the expanding numbers of very old people, but it may be that these older patients, who are mainly women, have a more normal lifespan than younger patients.

Multi-infarct dementia

The common belief that dementia is caused by 'hardening of the arteries' is in the majority of cases untrue. The blood supply to the brain was not mentioned when discussing the commoner cause, ATD. To the pathologist the blood vessels in ATD show some changes in their walls, but they are not narrowed by arteriosclerosis. It is possible using special scanning techniques to study the regional blood flow to various areas of the brain. These methods show a reduction in flow to those areas most affected in cases of ATD and particularly the frontal lobes, but this is likely to be due to the fact that when an area of brain becomes less active its blood supply automatically reduces; it is effect rather than cause. So, Alzheimer-type dementia is not due to 'hardening of the arteries'.

MID and general arteriosclerosis

However, it has been known for many years that, probably in about 20 to 30% of dementia sufferers, the primary cause of the dementia is connected with actual disease of the arteries. This condition was in the past called *arteriosclerotic dementia* or *vascular dementia* and it was generally assumed that the narrowing of arteries by arteriosclerosis reduced the amount of blood flowing to the brain as a whole and so gradually damaged its functions.

This concept had to be modified as the pathology of the condition became clearer and as newer techniques were developed to demonstrate blood flow to the brain. There is no doubt about the connection with disease of the blood vessels. These patients usually show other evidence of arteriosclerosis elsewhere in the body — heart disease, poor circulation to the legs, or, most commonly, high blood pressure. It has even been suggested that high blood pressure in a dementing person is proof that the cause of their dementia is vascular.

Infarcts. But it is not narrowing of the large blood vessels by arteriosclerosis and a consequent general reduction in blood flow to the whole brain that causes the damage to nerve cells. Rather, pathologists have shown, all over the cerebral cortex, multiple, very tiny areas of damage. In each of these areas the brain substance is softened. Under the microscope the cells are seen to be dead or degenerating. The local blood supply to each tiny area has been completely cut off by a small stroke — the blockage or rupture of a very small blood vessel that feeds that particular area. Sometimes the blockage is due to blood clots, called *emboli*, which travel from a distance, from the damaged walls of the bigger arteries in the head and neck, or from clots in the heart; sometimes the blockage develops locally by thrombosis or bleeding in the arteriosclerotic vessels, for reasons that are not yet entirely clear.

The area of dead brain tissue caused by such a blockage is called an *infarct* and the disorder has been renamed *multi-infarct dementia* (MID). If large enough the infarcts can be seen at certain stages in their development on a CT scan or by using a newer technique, nuclear magnetic resonance (NMR) scanning. Yet another new scanning technique called positron emission tomography (PET) can demonstrate what is happening to the general and local blood flow of the brain and how well blood oxygen and other nutrients are being used up. After a stroke causing an infarct in the brain, the PET scan shows that the blood supply to the brain tissue surrounding the dead area recovers quite quickly.

So multi-infarct dementia is caused by a combination of many little strokes; it is *linked* to the general disease of the blood vessels called arteriosclerosis, but is not due to generally reduced blood flow to the brain as a whole.

The course of MID

Understanding the pathology of MID helps us to understand how a patient with this condition declines mentally (Table 1.8).

Mass action. Firstly, the law of mass action applies. It has been shown that the total area of cerebral softening, adding together all the little areas of infarction, is proportional to the degree of intellectual impairment.

Irregular course. Secondly, the fact that these little infarcts occur repeatedly over a number of years is reflected in the course of the dementia (see Fig. 2.1). Usually it is quite difficult to chart when each little stroke happens, for the tiny changes are subtle and merge into each other. The result is a steady decline, just as in ATD. From time to time, however, a more dramatic change may occur and the decline becomes irregular or stepwise.

During an acute episode, just as with strokes not related to MID, the suddenness of the change and the disruption and swelling (oedema) around the infarct can lead to a more generalized, though temporary, disruption of brain function, called acute confusion (p. 44). The patient becomes noticeably more disoriented with 'clouding of consciousness', ranging from mild drowsiness to coma.

This acute confusion may begin to clear quite quickly as can happen to the physical after-effects of a stroke, for example a paralysis or speech problem. But sometimes confusion after a stroke can persist for weeks before it clears, and only then can we begin to see how much permanent damage there is.

A brief stroke episode, recovering within a few hours and

with no evidence of permanent damage, is called a *transient ischaemic attack.*

In contrast to these sudden changes, MID patients may also go through periods when their functional level remains fairly static, or even improves over weeks or months, for the brain can slowly reorganise its functions to some extent after an infarct, so long as no new damage occurs (see p. 42).

Patchy damage. Thirdly, though it is widespread, the damage is patchy, all over the brain. The strokes may hit one or other of those areas which serve very specific functions, the result being that the patient suffers, temporarily or permanently, an impairment of speech, or the paralysis of one side of the body, or partial blindness (hemianopia). Most of the strokes however will occur in areas with no specific function, the association or connecting areas of the brain.

The quite extensive areas of cortex *not* damaged by strokes can go on working relatively normally, though of course the connections between these and other areas may have been damaged. The result is that some general functions such as personality, or insight, or the ability to respond emotionally may not decline as much as, say, memory or speech.

Multi-infarct dementia can therefore be much more distressing to the patient than Alzheimer-type dementia, where the person's ability to respond is blunted and their insight is lost at roughly the same rate as the general decline.

Despite the patchiness and irregular progression of MID, however, the overall course of the illness is downwards and the decline may be just as steady and generalised as in ATD. At any stage, this course is likely to be complicated by disorders of the other arteries in the body — a coronary attack, problems related to hypertension, or of course a more major stroke. The cause of death in multi-infarct dementia is therefore likely to be one of these events rather than the gradual fading away of ATD.

Causes of MID

The cause of generalised arteriosclerosis is not yet clear. Diet and genetic factors play a part. More specifically it is not clear why a particular tiny vessel should block at a particular time and cause an area of brain to infarct and the cells around it to die. Only in the case of clots coming from other arteries — emboli — is the cause of the damage obvious.

Drugs for MID

There have been many attempts to use drugs to improve cerebral circulation. Theoretically such drugs are unlikely to help in MID, except possibly during the immediate aftermath of a stroke, for the blood supply to the rest of the brain appears to continue to function well or, if reduced, recovers quickly. In the area of an infarct the damage is permanent, the cells are dead and they cannot be revived. In practice it has been surprisingly difficult to show whether such drugs are effective, because the fluctuations and variability of MID make assessment of the results a complicated matter. The often contradictory results of a great many drug trials can be summarized by saying that, as yet, there has been no definite proof that a particular drug delays the progress of decline in MID.

Aspirin, dipyridamole and other drugs have been used in younger patients to prevent transient ischaemic attacks by reducing the formation of tiny emboli. This is a more hopeful approach which could lead to the development of preventative drugs which would lessen the frequency of the small strokes of MID and thus slow or halt the decline.

MID and ATD

Despite the differences in pathological changes and the differences in their detailed courses, it is very often quite difficult to tell a case of multi-infarct dementia from one of Alzheimer-type dementia. Furthermore, pathological studies show that there are many mixed cases with both diagnoses.

It is almost impossible to be sure in what proportion the two conditions occur, since demented patients may end their days in such a variety of places — home, nursing home, residential home or any of a variety of types of hospital — and it is therefore difficult to find a representative sample. One estimate is about 60 ATD cases to 20 MID cases to 20 mixed.

For practical purposes we will only be able to distinguish very definite, classical MID cases from very definite ATD

Table 1.8 Hachinski's score for the diagnosis of MID (adapted from
Hachinski V C et al 1975 Archives of Neurology 32:632)

Abrupt onset	2
Stepwise deterioration	1
Fluctuating course	2
Nocturnal confusion	1
Relative preservation of personality	1
Depression	1
Somatic complaints	1
Emotional lability	1
History of hypertension	1
History of stroke	1
Evidence of arteriosclerosis elsewhere	2
Focal neurological signs	2
Focal neurological symptoms	2
Total score possible	18

A score of more than 7 is said to favour the diagnosis of Multi-infarct
dementia.

cases, with considerable vagueness in between. At present
there is limited value anyway in making the distinction; the
only help that the information can be to patients or relatives
is to tell them either that in MID the decline is likely to be
erratic, with strokes and other evidence of arteriosclerosis, or
that in ATD it will be more gradual.

It is more important to make an accurate distinction for the
purposes of research, where it is essential to study as pure
as possible a sample of ATD or MID patients. The Hachinski
Score (Table 1.8) is one useful attempt to make the distinction
and, incidentally, provides a good summary of the special
features of multi-infarct dementia.

Other causes of dementia

The other possible causes of a gradual decline in brain function are many and they are all much less common (Table 1.5).
Probably no more than 5% of elderly patients with dementia
suffer from one or other of these rarer illnesses, though they
are relatively more common in younger patients. It has even
been suggested that as many as 15% of dementing patients
under the age of 70 have a remediable cause. Diagnostic

investigation is therefore more important in younger patients and in some cases leads on to effective treatment. However, the list of rarer causes includes some tragically untreatable illnesses.

Transmitter defect

Parkinsonism

Patients suffering from Parkinson's disease have been shown to be more likely than other people of the same age to suffer dementia. Perhaps 20% of parkinsonism patients are so affected. Parkinson's disease is chiefly a disorder of a nucleus of nerve cells, deep in the centre of the brain, called the substantia nigra. Because of the death of cells in this nucleus there is a reduction in the neurotransmitter dopamine, and this is what causes the typical symptoms. The dementia which parkinsonism patients develop, however, is thought to be due to reduction in acetylcholine, and there is evidence in affected patients of cell death in the nucleus of Meynert. So this dementia is quite like ATD, although it is probably not identical.

Physical damage

Normal pressure hydrocephalus

Relatively commoner in younger patients, this condition, in which the flow of cerebrospinal fluid inside the brain is partially or from time to time blocked, may follow quite a long time after head injuries, meningitis or neurosurgery, or may appear out of the blue. As a result of the blockage the ventricles of the brain swell but the brain substance itself cannot expand within the rigid skull box. If a 'shunt' is inserted by a neurosurgeon to take away excess fluid into the blood circulation, the function of the brain may recover, as long as the dementia has not progressed too far. It is certainly very worthwhile looking for this condition especially in younger patients and most especially when two particular symptoms occur at an early stage of the dementia — incontinence and inco-ordination of walking or other movements, called 'gait dyspraxia'.

Repeated head injury

If a person suffers repeated injuries to the brain, the law of mass action eventually operates and generalized impairment of the brain's function can occur, often together with other neurological abnormalities such as parkinsonism. This is of course commonest among boxers — the 'punch drunk' syndrome. Surprisingly, impairment occasionally only begins some time after the boxer finishes his career, suggesting that other factors, such as ordinary ageing, add to the damage to make the patient cross the 'threshold' of dementia.

Slowly growing tumours of the brain

Secondary tumours arising from a primary tumour elsewhere in the body, or a primary tumour of the coverings of the brain, a meningioma, which may grow very slowly, can lead to gradual mental impairment as they grow in the brain. Tumour is therefore another potentially treatable cause of the dementia syndrome.

Toxic damage

The most potent insidious external poison which can cause brain damage is lead, and fears that lead from petrol might be affecting the brain function of children have caused considerable public debate. Aluminium poisoning in dialysis patients has already been mentioned. Certain poisons can also reach toxic levels in the brain because of a failure to get rid of them from the body, for example copper levels are not controlled in the bodies of patients suffering from Wilson's disease and they may develop dementia at a young age. Wilson's disease is a genetic condition whose effects on the brain can be avoided by drug treatment.

Alcoholism

Chronic alcoholics often develop a specific recent memory loss called Korsakoff's syndrome (p. 55). This is progressive if the person continues to drink. If the patient stops drinking, the damage becomes static, or, as after a head injury or stroke, some recovery of function may be possible over months or even years. Since it does not affect the overall function of the cerebrum Korsakoff's syndrome is not strictly speaking a dementia. In addition to this syndrome, however, there is now evidence that some alcoholics develop a more generalized shrinking of the brain which shows up on CT scanning. It is likely that this shrinkage is a sign of a developing general dementia.

Genetic disorder

Huntington's chorea

This disorder develops mainly in the patient's 40s or 50s, though sometimes even earlier and sometimes later in life. The dementia is combined with a specific neurological sign — chorea, that is, dancing, jerky movements of the limbs. As well as the widespread damage of dementia there is also local damage to nuclei deep in the centre of the brain and it is this damage which leads to the involuntary movements. It is emerging that, as in Alzheimer-type dementia, there may be a decline in neurotransmitter systems in Huntington's chorea. In this case the transmitter involved in GABA (gamma-amino-butyric acid).

This illness is best known, however, because not only is it a genetic disorder like Wilson's disease, but it is very directly inherited by a dominant gene — one that always expresses itself in illness if a person inherits it. This means that if one parent suffers from the condition there is a 50% chance *at each birth* of the child having the gene and developing the condition. The consequences for families and the difficulties of genetic counselling will be discussed later (p. 192).

There has been considerable progress towards finding a 'genetic marker', something which shows whether a particular person carries the gene for Huntington's chorea or not. However, until we can be 100% sure that such markers are completely accurate in predicting whether a person has the gene or not, and until there is an effective preventative treatment of the condition their use for genetic counselling will be controversial.

Infections

General paralysis of the insane (GPI)

Historically this is the most important type of dementia, being the end stage of the 'scourge of Europe', syphilis, an untreatable condition until early this century. It usually starts 10–20 years after the initial infection if that was untreated. As well as the dementia, patients show other neurological signs. Despite treatment now being available for syphilis, occasional cases still occur and it is worth looking out for, since it is treatable if an antibiotic is given before the brain damage has become too severe. Whether the newer scourge of AIDS will lead to dementia in those who do not die early remains to be seen.

Creutzfeldt-Jakob disease

This extremely rare dementia, associated with other neurological signs, is interesting mainly because it has been linked with an almost identical disorder called Kuru, a type of dementia which used to be passed by cannibalism in New Guinea, and itself has been shown to pass from person to person, for example by corneal transplants from a dead sufferer. It is caused by so-called slow virus or a 'prion' (p. 20) and is at present untreatable.

Vitamin deficiencies

Deficiency of the vitamins niacin (causing pellagra), B12 and folic acid can all lead to forms of dementia which get better if the vitamins are replaced. Although simply treated these are uncommon causes of dementia.

Endocrine disorders

Disturbance of the parathyroid and thyroid hormones can lead to dementia which is treatable. Thyroid deficiency (hypothyroidism) is the commonest of these disorders, but unfortunately many patients suffer from both hypothyroidism *and* ATD and treatment of the one does not influence the other.

White matter damage

Multiple sclerosis

This, and indeed any condition which involves widespread patchy damage to the brain, can eventually lead by 'mass action' to a general decline. The dementia of multiple sclerosis is usually fairly mild, and is sometimes first noticed when the patient seems surprisingly bland emotionally in the face of their progressing disabilities. The damage in multiple sclerosis is caused by 'plaques' which develop in the white matter of the brain; the grey matter is not directly affected.

Binswanger's disease

Here again the white matter seems to be the site of the damage, so that the connecting nerve fibres of the brain are gradually interrupted and function gradually declines. Like MID, it is connected with arteriosclerosis. It is a new discovery, a variant of vascular dementia, but without the infarcts of MID. It is not yet known how common the condition is.

CONCLUSION

This list of causes of dementia is not exhaustive, and many of the types of dementia are quite rare. Nevertheless it is important, particularly in younger patients, to investigate the cause of dementia fully and to look for remediable conditions, and in older patients to keep in mind the rare possibility that something more curative can be achieved. Two illnesses, ATD and MID, remain the chief causes of the decline and disability of dementia.

2

What is not dementia?

Having defined what dementia *is*, the next step is to define what it is *not*. In other words, what other illnesses or states of mind can be mistaken for dementia? From our original definition (p. 1) we can see that:

— any condition which is not a decline from normal cannot
  be dementia
— any condition which is not gradually progressive cannot
  be dementia
— a decline affecting only one or two aspects of mental
  function cannot be dementia

This may seem like stating the obvious, but, as this chapter will show, looking at each of these statements in turn can help to clarify dementia and its boundaries. There are three good reasons for examining these boundaries closely.

Careless diagnosis

In the first place, there has been a tendency to be careless with the word dementia and this carelessness can have serious consequences. If it is assumed that an old lady's failure to cope at home is due to dementia, without considering other possible causes, she may be wrongly

34

placed in residential or hospital care, when, in fact, she is suffering from a simple physical condition or a different psychiatric disorder which could have easily been treated in her own home, or treated better in a different setting.

Likewise, this carelessness tempts doctors, brought up to look only on cure as success and seeing that dementia is largely incurable, to dismiss the demented from their attention, except as an increasing nuisance. Elderly patients in an acute medical ward who are labelled as 'demented' without adequate diagnosis or assessment of their problems may be put in the corner, as it were, to get a second class sort of treatment. If dementia is the right diagnosis, then their special needs are likely to be overlooked. If it is the wrong diagnosis, then their actual illness may go undiagnosed and untreated.

There are lesser versions of this hasty labelling. We do it when, as visitors to a residential home or geriatric hospital, we see all the residents in the day room as the same and assume that they are all 'confused old ladies'. There is an implication that everybody has the same problem and that that problem is dementia. The un-demented are treated as demented and all may be poorly treated.

Difficult diagnosis

A second reason for spending time on definition is that, with the best will in the world, being sure that a person actually suffers from dementia can be surprisingly difficult. This again has practical implications. We would like as early as possible in the illness to alert the patient and her relatives to the problems they will face in the future, and to teach them how best to cope with these problems. On the other hand, the diagnosis of dementia is an ominous one; if it is diagnosed wrongly or too early, unnecessary distress can be caused. Unfortunately, early *and* accurate diagnosis is not always possible.

Research diagnosis

The third reason to attempt a clear, exclusive definition concerns research. If it were possible to draw clear boundaries between what is and what is not dementia then we could study the dementing group as a whole, comparing it with the rest of the population or with groups of sufferers from other conditions. In this way we could find out much more about the specific causes and effects of dementia.

If such clear definition is not possible (and that is in effect how things stand at present) research is more difficult. We are only able to compare a group who are definitely dementing against a group who are not dementing. Other research then has to focus on the grey area between dementia and normality and on the grey area between dementia and other conditions. Is the boundary vague because good enough tests are not yet available in order to make clear distinctions; is it vague because there is actual overlap between the conditions, so that one merges into the order; or is it vague because there are other, intermediate conditions which complicate the picture?

We will touch on these points further as we now look again at the stages of our definitions to examine the '*differential diagnosis*' of dementia — what it is not.

DEMENTIA IS A DECLINE FROM NORMAL

Dementia and the normal changes of ageing

Dementia is not 'just old age'. In the first chapter I have outlined some of the evidence that distinguishes the *pathology* of the illnesses of dementia from normal changes in the ageing brain. In practical terms how can we make this distinction?

Let us firstly look at what normal psychological changes occur in old age; then we can compare these with the changes of dementia (Table 2.1). This is difficult, however, because one of the chief characteristics of older people as a group is the huge range of their mental and physical capacities. Different individuals seem to age at different rates; and different aspects of each particular person's bodily and mental functions seem to age at different rates. Furthermore, each individual and each function have begun the changes of old age from widely different normal levels in earlier life.

So it is quite difficult to decide what is normal and what is

Table 2.1 Psychological changes in normal old age and in dementia

Normal ageing	Dementia
Slowing	More severe and increasing
Cautiousness	Variable
Reduced ability to solve new problems	More severe and increasing
Disengagement?	Variable
Mildly impaired memory?	More severe and increasing
Mildly impaired intelligence?	More severe and increasing

abnormal in the ageing mind. Even trying to follow change in one individual over the decades of old age is difficult, for many factors complicate the interpretation of tests of intelligence, memory and other brain functions.

Slowing

Some changes are clear and almost universal. The most striking one is a slowing down of both physical and mental activity. Indeed, this change will be obvious to anybody who is over the age of 40, though it probably begins as early as our 20s. It becomes more and more obvious as we enter old age.

The slowing in reactions affects our ability to perform any test which requires speed, for example, many intelligence tests. It is a source of frustration to the many older people who miss the ability to be quick off the mark, and an annoyance to quicker younger people who become impatient with their elders. One of the first lessons which anybody caring for an old person has to learn is that they must slow down to a speed that allows the older person to work with them.

When older people complain that they are becoming 'confused', they are sometimes referring to this slowness in their interactions with younger people, and the resulting feeling of being rushed.

An exaggeration of the mental showing of old age is a prominent feature of dementia (p. 111). It is possible to measure reaction time to a variety of stimuli and show that this is greatly delayed in moderately or severely demented patients; but, as with other mental changes in dementia, it is extremely difficult to define the boundary between *normal* slowing and this *excessive* and *progressive* slowing.

Rigidity and disengagement

Another frequently noted change of old age is an increasing abhorrence of the new-fangled. Although it is true that some old people are as adventurous (or as fickle) as adolescents exploring their life, their emotions and relationships for the first time, for many, old age is a time of regularity, order and sameness.

To some extent this may come about because both young people and old people expect it to be so. But there does seem to be a natural biological change towards rigidity. The ageing brain may not be so able to adjust to new patterns of experience; it may not be so flexible as in young people. The result is that older people tend to be more cautious when new things occur, tend to have difficulty learning new concepts and activities and tend to prefer a routine existence.

The older person may well feel quite comfortable doing very little for long periods. In the past this 'dis-engagement' from activity has had its advantages. The elder has been a stable focus for family life. Distance from the hurly-burly, coupled with a lifetime's experience, could allow elders to be wiser than their rash young relatives. With greater social mobility and an increase in the numbers of old people, this traditional role has been challenged. Older people are nowadays not so likely to be in a stable social position for the rest of their lives. They may need to make quite major and dramatic decisions about where they live, or need to develop new relationships and interests which must last for many years of retirement or widowhood.

The normal mental changes of old age do not help in these crises and many an old person clings to the limited life that they have, instead of facing up to the need to be adventurous and explore in order to obtain satisfaction in life. Once again in dementia there is a gross and progressive exaggeration of this rigidity and difficulty with new situations (p. 111).

Intellectual functions

When it comes to memory (p. 101), intellect (p. 111) and all the other higher mental functions which decline so obviously in dementia it is surprisingly uncertain to what extent these functions change during normal old age. As I have indicated, many people interpret the slowness of old age as a decline in intellect. Moreover, when intelligence tests are given in the right circumstances, allowing for the older person's slowness and cautiousness, they show remarkably little general decline till very old age. There is argument about memory impairment too. Probably some of the complex aspects of processing memories do decline in old age, but never as severely as in dementia.

It is strange then that nearly one-half of a surveyed group of people over 75 complained of memory impairment, whereas we know that probably 75% or more of them are mentally entirely normal (Table 1.1). The statistic is stranger still when we consider that if there *were* dementia sufferers in the group some of them might well not realize that their memory was impaired, and so would *not* complain.

Who are the 25% or more who complained of memory impairment but were not in fact impaired? Some must have been noticing the normal changes of old age and were worried by them. Some may have been suffering from other illnesses or the effects of drugs which made them feel mentally dulled or actually confused. Some may have been feeling distressed for other reasons, but interpreted their distress as mental impairment (p. 58).

Differentiating from dementia

What then can we say to an older person who thinks that she may be losing her memory, that is, developing dementia; or to her family who are worried that she is declining mentally?

Likelihood of dementia

Firstly, we need to ask carefully why they are worried at this particular time, because quite separate events or concerns may be on their minds.

Then we can look at the statistics and see that the chances of dementia occurring in a particular individual are actually quite low, maybe one in four or five if they survive into their 80s. This statistic is, of course, of little reassurance to an individual.

If the concern has arisen because one of the patient's own parents or a brother or sister suffered dementia we can look at the genetic statistics, but once again these are of little individual help. We can merely say that, on average, there is only a minor hereditary component to dementia, so that the risk is still fairly small, though it is bigger than if there had not been a close relative who suffered dementia.

Pattern and degree of change

It is more important to look at how the complaint has developed over time (Fig. 2.1). Dementia is a new development, a decline at a much greater rate than anything that could be the result of normal ageing. If we can get a history of how well the patient was functioning previously — her baseline level — we can work out the pattern of decline. But, even with a good baseline, change will only be obvious over many months. Nevertheless, this is the best way of ensuring proper diagnosis.

When someone is severely demented there is, of course, little doubt about the diagnosis. Although some of the changes resemble normal old age the *degree* of change is far beyond what would normally occur.

And, in fact, some of the symptoms of dementia, such as disinhibition, dysphasia, dyspraxia, incontinence, never occur in normal older people (though they may occur in *other* illnesses that are common in old age).

At the earliest stages there is, however, no test which will clearly distinguish the normal person from the dementing person. Indeed, many patients who appear to be developing dementia, and perform rather badly on tests of memory or intelligence, actually seem to improve on later testing, so it can be dangerous to make the diagnosis too early.

The correct action is to 'wait and see', a very uncertain position for both patient and family to be in. The uncertainty can be tempered by reassurance that the patient will be reviewed later and that, if necessary, help will then be available. This should not stop us from trying to assess dementia sufferers as early as possible. For early assessment can rule out other causes of the patient's apparent decline, and helps to provide the baseline from which it is easier to see at a later

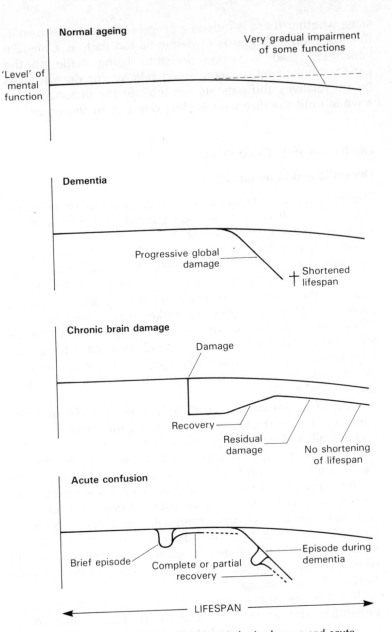

Fig. 2.1 The time course of dementia, chronic brain damage and acute confusion, compared to normal ageing.

stage whether there is indeed a progressive dementia or not. But fixing on a diagnosis of dementia too early is a mistake which can lead to wrong decisions being made on the patient's behalf by overconcerned relatives or doctors. It is best if relatives and patients can tolerate the uncertainty for a while until the diagnosis is clear one way or the other.

DEMENTIA IS PROGRESSIVE

Dementia and brain damage

The decline of dementia can be relatively fast or relatively slow, but in all patients it is progressive; the patient is always on a downward slope (Fig. 2.1).

For a particular patient the decline will not always continue at an even rate. Occasionally ATD patients have long static spells in between periods of more rapid decline. In addition, the downward course is often modified, as we have seen, in MID, where repeated strokes occur throughout the illness. At each of these strokes there may be a sudden deterioration followed by a static period, or even a temporary improvement. But there are very many such episodes and the general impression, taken over months and years, is still of progressive decline.

Now, if a person has had only *one* episode of brain damage, say one stroke, or a head injury, the damage is once and for all and will not progress further (Fig. 2.1). Indeed, although the damaged brain's *structure* cannot be repaired in the way a skin wound repairs, the brain can reorganise its connections to some extent so that over a few months, or sometimes 1 or 2 years, some recovery of *function* is possible and improvement occurs. Eventually that recovery is as complete as it can be. From then on, for the rest of that persons's life, there will be a residual degree of brain damage which is *static*. Table 2.2 gives a list of some of the possible causes of brain damage.

The 'law of mass action' (p. 10) applies here as in dementia. The greater the volume of brain damaged or destroyed, the greater the loss of general functions such as intelligence, long-term memory, abstract thinking, and reasoning. So there might be justification in describing a

Table 2.2 Some causes of chronic (non-progressive) brain damage

Head injury	
Brain surgery	
Cerebrovascular accident	Stroke
	Embolus
	Intracerebral haemorrhage
	Subarachnoid haemorrhage
Infection	Encephalitis
	Meningitis

severely but now statically brain-damaged patient as demented, but they are not going through the process of dementia, they are not dement*ing*. Using the term dementia at all here can be misleading. If we use the term '*chronic brain damage*', implying a permanent condition, we describe exactly what has happened and can expect that characteristic slow but limited improvement.

There are intermediate cases between dementia proper and what I have called chronic brain damage. If a person suffers a *few* strokes, but with long intervals between them, then during those long intervals her progress will follow the rules of brain damage. But each ensuing stroke adds to the previous damage so that overall her impairment gets worse and worse. Neither term is quite appropriate here, and either will do.

Treatable or reversible dementia

Some illnesses follow the course of dementia only as long as their particular cause is present (see Table 1.5) and so are intermediate between brain damage and dementia in another way. The punch-drunk boxer may stop getting worse when he stops boxing and may even recover a little over the next few years to be left with residual permanent damage (but not always — see p. 30). Likewise, surgery for hydrocephalus or a brain tumour can halt the progress of dementia. The patient with syphilis who develops GPI continues to decline mentally till antibiotic treatment is given and then may recover well if the damage has not been too severe.

Potentially, if we could treat ATD, MID, or the other rarer

causes, they also could be added to the list of partly or wholly reversible dementias. It is therefore quite reasonable for the present to describe patients who have treatable causes as dement*ing* while the cause continues progressively to damage their brains, and then as chronically brain damaged if, after the cause is removed, the damage becomes static.

Dementia and mental handicap

When dementia begins, the sufferer's brain has been in its adult developed state for many years. In mental handicap, however, the brain is damaged at a stage when it is still maturing and developing. There are some parallels between the brain damage/dementia distinction and the two principal types of mental handicap.

In the first type an episode of brain damage before or around the time of birth leaves a static amount of residual impairment. The brain still has some capacity to mature and develop, though now limited by the damage. The child does develop mentally but lags behind other children. This then is a form of chronic brain damage. The other type of mental handicap is more like dementia. For example, some metabolic disorders lead to the deposition of more and more of a toxic chemical in the brain, causing progressive impairment. This counteracts the process of maturation, so that the child declines and dies.

Dementia and acute confusion

If dementia can be seen as a *gradual* failure of the workings of the brain, then acute confusion is *rapid* failure (in all medical terminology 'acute' means rapid in onset and brief in duration). Like dementia, acute confusion is a *syndrome*. It can be caused by anything which rapidly damages the brain as a whole — direct damage to the brain by injury or disease; general illnesses which disturb brain function; or poisons and drugs which affect the brain (Table 2.3).

Reversibility. The importance of recognising acute confusion comes from the fact that, if the disease or damage that is causing it can be treated or stops spontaneously, the acute confusion will clear. Confusion is not progressive unless the

Table 2.3 Some causes of acute confusion

Direct damage to the brain	Head injury Cerebrovascular accident (thrombosis, embolus or haemorrhage) Subdural haemorrhage after injury Epileptic fit (post-ictal) Postoperative Infection (meningitis, encephalitis) Sudden change in a brain tumour
General disorders which disturb brain function	Constipation (reason unclear) Infection (especially chest or urinary tract) Cardiac failure and other heart disorders Kidney failure (raised blood urea) Liver failure Respiratory failure (raised carbon dioxide) Vitamin deficiency (lack of thiamin — vitamin B1 — in alcoholics) Endocrine disorders (especially hypoglycaemia in diabetics)
Drugs	Tranquillizers including alcohol Antidepressants Antiparkinsonian drugs Digoxin and other cardiac drugs Cimetidine (for peptic ulcers) and many others
Drug withdrawal	Alcohol (delirium tremens — DTs) Benzodiazepines (including diazepam and lorazepam) Barbiturates

Acute confusion due to any cause is more likely to occur in young children, the elderly and dementia sufferers.

cause is progressive. On the other hand, if the cause is very severe or very progressive, it will take the patient past the stage of confusion to coma or even death. Acute confusion is therefore a medical problem, requiring accurate diagnosis and treatment of its cause as a matter of urgency, with hope of recovery.

Terminology. The word *confusion* is, unfortunately, 'confusing' in itself. It has been used to mean muddled thinking, disorientation, clouding of consciousness, or the whole syndrome of acute confusion, and is even regularly used to mean dementia (as in 'the confused elderly'). It should be avoided where possible, or only used to mean 'the syndrome of acute confusion'. Even better would be to use other terms, such as *acute cerebral failure, acute brain failure* or *acute brain syndrome*. Older terms like *delirium* and *toxic confusion* as well as these newer terms refer to exactly the same syndrome.

Course

Figure 2.2 shows the course of acute confusion after damage to the brain. It may take hours, or even days, to develop after the cause begins. Sometimes there is a *retrograde amnesia*, the patient losing memories from shortly before the time the confusion started. Thus she may not recall the fall, or taking the extra pills, or the beginnings of a chest infection which caused her confusion. Confusion reaches a maximum level if the cause is not progressive and will begin to recover after the cause is removed.

However, this recovery can be delayed for quite a long time, particularly in very elderly people or people who suffer from dementia. For example, a case of delirium tremens (DTs), the acute confusion which can occur when an alcoholic cuts down their intake of alcohol rapidly, can, in an elderly person, last several weeks before recovery begins. A patient who develops acute confusion after a stroke may likewise remain confused for weeks and then recover (in contrast, *physical* recovery after a stroke usually begins quite soon or not at all). So we can hope that a patient will make a quick recovery from acute confusion, but should not be surprised if it takes longer.

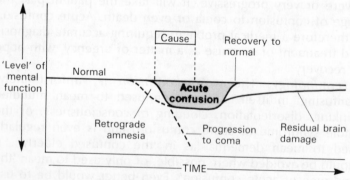

Fig. 2.2 The course of acute confusion.

Outcome

The *degree* of recovery which eventually occurs depends on two factors. First, what was the previous state of the patient? If she was not suffering from dementia we can hope that she will return to normal. Often, however, the patient with acute confusion was already dementing (Fig. 2.1), and her best possible recovery is to her previous degree of dementia.

The other factor is whether or not the damage to the brain is permanent (Fig. 2.2). If it is extensive enough or prolonged enough then, after the acute phase, there will be some degree of residual brain damage. The patient will not return to her previous normal but will be left with intellectual or other deficits of brain function, which then follow the course of brain damage as described on page 42.

Acute confusion during dementia

Acute confusion seems particularly common among dementia sufferers. This is partly because so many of them are very elderly anyway, and are therefore prone to develop all sorts of other illnesses and drug reactions which can cause confusion. Self-neglect and forgetfulness will increase the chances of such problems occurring. Perhaps also we notice acute confusion more in dementing people because they are so often in care. But in addition they have often no other way of complaining. For, instead of the limited retrograde amnesia mentioned above, a dementing person may have no memory at all of the recent past (p. 104). Furthermore she may not be fully aware of where a pain is or what she feels wrong or may have difficulty describing symptoms (p. 114).

The result is that, especially for more severely demented people, just as for children before they can talk, the only evidence that they are ill is either that they look ill or that they develop acute confusion. This makes it doubly important that families and staff caring for dementing people know a little about acute confusion and are on the look out for any rapid change that occurs. Doctors need to know that when such a change happens it means that something medical is wrong, and that if they can diagnose and treat the cause then the patient is likely to recover to her previous level.

Differentiating from dementia

The importance of being able to tell the difference between dementia and acute confusion, or being able to tell when a dementing person develops acute confusion on top of their dementia, is clear. How can we do this (Table 2.4)?

Table 2.4 Differentiating acute confusion and dementia

Acute confusion	Dementia
Rapid onset	Slowly progressive
Acute medical cause	Slowly progressive cause
Clouding of consciousness	Clear consciousness
Sleep disturbance	Normal sleep, but 'clock' may be wrong
Irregular variability	Tends to be worse towards evening, otherwise stable
Restlessness and unease	Settled apart from aimless wandering or searching
Visual hallucinations	Hallucinations uncommon and not usually disturbing
Emotional lability and distress	Poverty of mood commoner, some are labile

Time scale

Dementia is slowly progressive. Acute confusion is acute, beginning as a rapid change over minutes, hours or days, not months or years. Because of retrograde amnesia and the general disruption of memory and thinking which are part of an acute confusional state the patient is not always able to describe this rapid change. We need information from a relative or someone else who has seen the patient regularly over the last few months.

Cause

Often the evidence of a cause is obvious — an infection, the physical effects of a stroke, a head injury; often it will not be so obvious. The commonest missed cause of all is constipation, but many of the other causes in Table 2.3 are difficult to detect and the patient may not be able to make the appropriate complaint. The situation is further complicated by the fact that in some people a very minor cause may lead to quite severe confusion; in others there may be more than one cause (e.g. an infection and alcohol abuse, or heart failure and the tablets given to treat it); whilst in yet others a potential cause of confusion may not actually be causing confusion (e.g. the dementing person who is unaffected mentally by a chest infection).

Clinical features

There are many similarities between the effects of slowly progressive brain failure — dementia — and acute brain failure — acute confusion. In both conditions the basic ability of the brain to make complicated connections is impaired. In both, therefore, the sufferer will not be able to organise thinking properly, will become disoriented and will be impaired in her ability to lay down, store or recall memories. All her higher mental functions will be affected. But even when the timescale is unclear, and even when a cause is not obvious, it is possible to make a good guess that mental impairment is acute rather than chronic from the symptoms and signs of impairment (Table 2.4). Acute damage to the brain seems to affect its workings in a different way to chronic damage. The main difference relates to consciousness.

Consciousness. Our level of consciousness, that is, how aware we are, how able to focus attention, how awake, is controlled largely by a switching mechanism in the middle of the brain, called the *reticular activating system*. It is this mechanism which wakes us or puts us to sleep, and which switches the brain into active attention when, for example, someone calls our name. In acute confusional states this system appears to be damaged, usually temporarily. If severely damaged, unconsciousness results. So acute confusion can be thought of as a sort of 'semi-coma'. The patient is drowsy or dopey, she cannot fix her attention and thinking becomes muddled.

Sleep. The switching mechanism of *sleep* is also disturbed in acute confusion. The patient may sleep for a longer, or for a shorter, period than usual, or never. She may be awake by night and asleep by day. Her sleep may be lighter than normal or disturbed by dreams and nightmares. She may be unclear as to what is real and what is a dream.

The dementing patient, on the other hand, is usually clear

mentally, in the sense that she is alert and fully awake when awake and normally asleep when asleep. However, if she happens to go to bed early, she may rise after her normal length of sleep ready for action at 1 a.m., for many older people do not require as much sleep as younger people so that 4 or 6 hours may be quite a 'normal' sleep, inconvenient as it is for family, neighbours or staff. The dementing patient has simply got the timing of her internal clock wrong, not the mechanism of sleep.

Variability. A striking feature of these impairments of consciousness is their variability. Now, both dementing and acutely confused people tend to become more disoriented in the evening and night-time (p. 90). The reason for this is not clear. Much of it is probably due to sensory deprivation — at night there are fewer visual and sound clues to help us find our bearings, but fatigue or other effects on the daily rhythms of the body may play a part. In acute confusion, however, there is often a much more irregular and unpredictable variation. From hour to hour or from minute to minute, even within the course of a sentence the patient may move from drowsiness to alertness, from disorientation to complete orientation, from muddled to clear thinking. This type of variability is unusual in a dementing person. Presumably it is caused by varying damage to the consciousness switch of the reticular system.

Restlessness. Also affected by this variability is another common feature of the acute confusional state — restlessness. By restlessness is meant an inability to settle both physically and mentally (a frequent accompaniment of physical illness even without actual confusion). The dementing person is not usually restless in this sense of suffering listlessness and unease. That may come as a surprise to those who work with dementing people in care, but it should be recalled that the majority of sufferers are quietly living at home or settled in care. Most of the restlessness which does occur in dementia appears aimless, or is understandable as a search for familiar surroundings. The restlessness of acute confusion is more like the result of physical discomfort or of mental distress.

Visual perception. Yet another feature of the acute confusional state (and one which in itself can lead to restlessness) is disturbance of visual perception. The patient misinterprets what she actually sees (visual *illusions*) or sees things that are not there are at all (visual *hallucinations*). Thus, she may see faces distorted, or strange colours, or faces in an empty window — all very bewildering or frightening experiences. Illusions and hallucinations are sometimes experienced in the other senses, for example, hearing (auditory) or smell (olfactory), but visual disturbances are by far the commonest. The reason for these disturbances is not clear. Perhaps there is impairment of another function of the reticular system, namely that of filtering out irrelevant information, which is part of the process of focusing attention (see p. 124).

Lability. Finally, the acutely confused patient's *emotions* are likely to be disturbed. As can be imagined, hallucinations and illusions upset the patient and may lead her to believe that someone is out to harm her — she believes that the devil is in the house, or that the nurses are having noisy parties in her ward and are singing rude songs about her, or that the police are after her. It is natural in these circumstances to feel fearful or angry. Furthermore the experience of disorientation is bewildering and frightening in itself. But as well as this the patient's *control* of her emotions may be lost, so that she finds herself suddenly losing her temper, or suddenly in tears, or suddenly laughing for no very clear reason, just as quickly regaining control. Her emotions may fluctuate like this (emotional 'lability') throughout the period of confusion or for a time she may get 'stuck' in a particular emotion, be it depression or anger or fear.

On the other hand, in dementia, although lability is not uncommon (p. 134), most sufferers show a more obvious decline or 'poverty' of emotion (p. 112).

Partial symptoms

All these clinical features are very common in people who are acutely confused, but they are not *all* always present. For a start the variability of confusion means that a person may appear clear at one time of the day and very confused at another. This can lead to problems in convincing doctors or senior care staff that a patient is acutely ill at all. A lady who is apparently clear for 90% of the day, but for short periods at night becomes drowsy, hallucinating and restless, is suffering from an acute confusional state, even if she can apparently answer all questions of orientation and memory perfectly during her clear spells (in reality it is likely that she will show patchy loss of memory and slight difficulty with complicated thinking most of the time, but these defects can be very difficult to pick up).

But it is not just this variability which leads to difficulty in diagnosing an acute confusional state. Only one or two of the characteristic signs may be evident in a particular patient. A lady with dementia may show no other change except that one day she begins to experience hallucinations, another merely develops sleep disturbance, yet these changes are enough evidence to diagnose acute confusion, call for the doctor, and ask what the cause is.

An everyday condition. Indeed, most of us have experienced some degree of acute confusion at some time. The person with influenza who feels a bit dopey and restless during the day and sleepless by night is suffering acute confusion, due to the effects of the 'flu virus on their brain function. And the person recovering from even a mild head injury or an operation who cannot think clearly for a while and asks what time it is (disorientation in time), where they are (disorientation in place) and what has been happening (memory impairment) is acutely confused.

Management of acute confusion

Find the cause and treat it. Acute confusion is thus a very common condition. Knowing its course, its distinguishing features and its possible causes, it should be possible for most people who help in looking after elderly people to differentiate someone suffering acute confusion from someone with dementia. The logical next step should be obvious. The cause of the acute confusion should be diagnosed as soon as possible (Table 2.3). The commonest causes are constipation, chest and urinary infections and drug side-effects or mistakes. Causes which are often missed include falls causing head injury and concussion; haemorrhage in the tissues covering the brain following a head injury (subdural haematoma) which can lead to a prolonged and often very variable confusion; fits; and delirium tremens, which can occur in alcoholics of all ages.

It is seldom necessary to look too far for the cause of confusion, for 'common things are common', but acute confusion does demand medical assessment. Sadly some of the causes are not treatable, the commonest of these being a stroke. During the course of a multi-infarct dementia, short or prolonged episodes of acute confusion may occur after each of a series of strokes. Despite the fact that such episodes are untreatable in themselves, they nevertheless need medical assessment.

Help with disorientation and hallucinations. Much of what will be said later about the management of disorientation and memory impairment in dementia (see Ch. 4) applies equally to people who are acutely confused. Special support at night is important, for that is when the confusion is likely to be at its worst. It is generally found that darkness increases disorientation and encourages hallucinations. A lighted room, with familiar objects and people around, is better.

If a patient experiences hallucinations and realises that they are imaginary, it is important to reassure her that she is not 'going mad', but that they will disappear when she is physically better. If she believes the hallucinations to be real, then it is of no value to get into an argument about their existence; it is more helpful to reassure her that she is actually seeing these things, but that they will eventually go away, and that in the meantime everything is being done to help get rid of them.

Help with distress. Confused patients are susceptible to the 'emotional temperature' around them and may misinterpret this in the same way that they misinterpret what they see and hear. A calm atmosphere, with the situation explained slowly, clearly and repeatedly, will help to prevent the patient from misunderstanding what is happening, and so lessen her distress. The worst possible place for an acutely confused patient is, unfortunately, the casualty department of a busy hospital, for its confusing bustle invites agitation and misinterpretation of the surroundings. The best place is her own home.

Indeed some elderly people, and especially elderly

dementing people, develop a sort of acute confusion just because of a move from one place to another — confusion of *translocation*. This may amount to a temporary disorientation when familiar surroundings are missed, or it may be a full blown acute confusional state. We should therefore be wary of moving elderly people around too much, especially if they are physically ill or suffering from dementia. The move itself can cause as much trouble as the reason for the move. Unfortunately, it is not possible to predict exactly who will be affected by a move in this way and who will be unaffected.

Drugs. Calmness, reassurance and orientation can be very helpful, but even so, for some patients, the combination of restlessness, emotional lability, bewildering confusion and frightening hallucinations is such that they are very disturbed, either panicking or aggressive. Drug treatment is therefore occasionally necessary, but it should always be borne in mind that among the list of causes of confusion are the very drugs which might be used to treat it (Table 2.3).

If anything is necessary, a night sedative may be used to help ease the worst time of confusion and lessen fatigue. By day, the smallest dose of tranquillizer that is necessary to prevent severe distress or aggression, or nothing at all, should be used. The only exceptions to this are for the acute confusion of delirium tremens (DTs) and during withdrawal from other tranquillizers such as diazepam or barbiturate drugs. In these conditions fits may occur along with the confusional state and it is often necessary to give an anti-epileptic tranquillizer, such as chlordiazepoxide, to prevent the fits.

Avoid long-term decisions. When a dementing patient, or even more especially an undemented person develops an acute confusional state, it is the wrong time to make major long-term decisions. Too often the acutely confused person lands in a general hospital bed because carers at home or in a residential home feel that they cannot cope. Once in the hospital the confusion caused by the move and the anxieties of carers lead to the inevitable decision that the patient cannot return home, even if there is little or no residual brain damage.

It is quite understandable that the carers should feel unable to cope during the disturbed period. They need outside support on an acute basis — a rapid response to an acute illness; and the patient requires adequate medical attention, diagnosis and treatment. General practitioners may need to be able to call on specialist hospital services, who will see the patient at home or at the outpatient clinic, so that *they* can feel supported if they wish to treat the confused patient at home.

If supportive home care services and adequate medical back-up were available we could hope that this short-term disorder could be managed without too much disruption to the patient's life, and that as a consequence long-term decisions could be made more sensibly after the acute confusion is over. If the patient has indeed suffered permanent brain damage new decisions *will* have to be made about her future support and care. If, however, she has returned to normal it is simply a time to reassess the pre-existing level of support.

DEMENTIA AFFECTS MOST ASPECTS OF MENTAL FUNCTION

Dementia and Korsakoff's syndrome

The fact that the dementias affect nerve cells and their connections over wide areas of the cerebral cortex means that widespread functions of the cortex are affected. Korsakoff's syndrome is also a progressive disorder but it only affects a small area of the brain, including the recent memory system of the hippocampal region (Fig. 1.2). It is not, therefore, a true dementia.

Recent memory loss and confabulation. Korsakoff's syndrome occurs mostly in alcoholics after years of heavy drinking, probably as a result of brain damage caused by deficiency of the vitamin thiamine (vitamin B1). Since it only affects this one area of the brain, the chief result of the damage is an impairment of recent memory. The sufferer often tries to compensate by *confabulation* (making up answers to cover gaps in the memory), which may be either conscious or automatic. Such confabulation is not, however, confined to Korsakoff patients (p. 182). It can occur in anyone who loses her memory, though it may be more elaborate in an alcoholic who has been used to telling tales about her drinking for many years.

Recovery. Korsakoff's syndrome is progressive if the patient goes on drinking, but its progress halts if she stops. It then follows the natural history of brain damage (p. 42) as long as she remains abstinent. Most doctors give thiamine supplements for some time in the hope that this will also help, though there is no clear evidence that it improves matters once the damage is done.

Dementia. Apart from the decline in memory most of the rest of the Korsakoff patient's brain is functioning normally. Their personality, intellect and old memories are all pretty well intact so they cannot be said to suffer dementia. However, they usually lack insight into the memory loss, and are often apathetic and repetitive. Indeed there may turn out to be quite an overlap between Korsakoff's syndrome and alcoholic dementia (p. 30), but until we know more about the latter condition, it is better to keep the distinction between them.

Pick's disease

Like Korsakoff's syndrome, this is a progressive but localized disorder. The damage is mainly to the frontal lobes of the brain (Fig. 1.2) with sometimes a little damage to the front of the temporal lobe as well. The main effect is a progressive decline in the patient's self-control (see Ch. 5), so that the personality deteriorates without any intellectual or memory loss. Sufferers seem to lose their conscience and moral sense, their ability to plan and to a greater or lesser extent their insight into their condition, but they are otherwise unchanged from normal.

The cause of Pick's disease is not known and there is no known treatment. Luckily it is a very rare condition but a particularly devastating one, for it affects mainly people in middle life. Furthermore, because all their intellectual capacities are preserved, they themselves usually think they are acting normally, whereas in fact they may be sexually disinhibited or irresponsible in decision-making, or their emotions may be out of their normal control. The result is that a previously responsible person may be causing social havoc but does not seem to care.

Distinguishing from dementia. Frontal lobe damage can occur in other conditions and is of course part of the overall damage of dementia (see Ch. 5). But when it is part of a dementia it usually has less impact than the blatant misbehaviour of a patient with Pick's disease. In some cases of multi-infarct dementia the strokes occur mostly in the frontal lobe and the patient may behave rather like a patient with Pick's disease, but there are usually a few other signs of generalized arteriosclerosis or of strokes elsewhere in the brain. In the same way trauma and brain tumours can cause a 'frontal lobe syndrome'. Pick's disease itself is in fact a rarity and all these other causes of frontal lobal damage are much more common.

PSEUDO-DEMENTIA

The conditions mentioned so far differ from dementia in important ways. We now come to a condition which may be indistinguishable from dementia. We already have a list of causes of reversible or treatable dementia (Table 1.5). These conditions have sometimes been labelled 'pseudo-dementia', but it is more accurate to stick to the term 'reversible dementia' where we think that the symptoms and signs of an *actual* dementia are caused by an illness which is slowly damaging the brain but can be treated. We would then only use the term pseudo-dementia to refer to the situation where the symptoms and signs of dementia are present but there is *no* actual damage to the brain; the patient behaves *as if* she were dementing but she is not in fact dementing. There is one principal cause of this pseudo-dementia — depressive illness.

Depressive illness

Severe depression is quite a common condition among elderly people, probably nearly as common as it is in people of middle age. I am not referring to the often mild, understandable depression which can follow one or other of the many loses which older people experience (and remember that dementia can be one of those losses — see p. 174). I am referring instead to those depressions whose severity is quite out of proportion to any precipitating loss (indeed, there is sometimes no obvious precipitant at all).

All the patient's activities and interests succumb to a slowing down and an all-pervading gloom. Usually the beginning of such a depression is fairly clear and the main complaints are the feeling of depression, a preoccupation with self-blame, guilt or hypochondriacal ideas, loss of interest (including loss of interest in food with consequent weight loss), loss of concentration, poor sleep with early wakening and a general slowing both physically and mentally.

However, sometimes in depression this mental slowing, together with poor concentration, loss of interest, social withdrawal and self-neglect, produces a state of detachment from the surrounding world which looks just like dementia. The patient appears to be disorientated, cannot concentrate and so cannot remember, and seems to have lost the ability to care for herself. On all the usual tests of intelligence, memory and orientation she may perform as if she were dementing. She may even *believe* that she is dementing — a variant of the hypochondriasis that is so often part of depression in older people. Perhaps some pseudo-dementia in depressive illness is caused by the patient acting out this belief, as if to prove her worst fears. If the onset of the illness has been slow, then it can be very easy to agree with her and conclude that she suffers from dementia.

Distinguishing from dementia

It is vital to distinguish patients with pseudo-dementia from those who are truly dementing, for they can usually be treated either by anti-depressant drugs or by ECT, and will make a good recovery after rehabilitation back to their normal activities. Among the many apparent dementia sufferers, how are we to pick out this particular group?

Hints of normality. Firstly, there may be hints that the 'dementia' is not as it should be. The patient maintains beneath her depression a normally active mind. So she may, to our surprise, register and recall the memory of one or two recent events which a dementing person would be expected to forget.

Symptoms of depression. Secondly, she is likely to complain of depression, or if not actually complaining, to look and act depressed. In particular, she may show the loss of appetite and weight loss characteristic of severe depression, and family or friends may have noted the striking slowing down ('retardation') of depression.

Diurnal variation. Thirdly, one of the characteristic features of depressive illness is that it tends to be worse in the morning, with early morning wakening, so that the patient's mood and activity improve as the day goes on. As we will see (p. 90), dementing patients function *worse* as the day progresses. A 'demented' patient who consistently livens up and becomes mentally clearer as the day progresses may not be demented at all but may have a treatable depression.

These observations and information gained from relatives or friends about how, when and what changes have occurred in the patient give us hints that the dementia is 'pseudo-' and that anti-depressant treatment should be tried.

Special tests. Many attempts have been made to find a test which will distinguish clearly between depression with pseudo- dementia and true organic dementia. Psychological tests, brain scans, EEG, and biochemical tests have all been tried. Unfortunately, none has yet been successful. There is too much overlap between the results, some dementing people scoring high on tests of depression and some depressed people scoring high on tests of dementia. Such overlaps make it impossible to interpret these tests in a particular individual.

Recovery. In general, it is worth erring on the side of optimism and starting treatment (though remaining cautious, as many anti-depressants are potent causes of confusion — Table 2.3). It can be extremely gratifying to see someone who was thought to be dementing make a complete recovery, particularly if plans had been made for her long-term care. And it can be pleasantly surprising when tests which have seemed to show dementia return to normal after treatment.

Other psychiatric disorders

Other disorders have frequently been mistaken for dementia, but this should really not occur, since the central feature of dementia is not present — the progressive decline in all mental functions. However, so prevalent is the notion that most or all mental illness or oddity in the elderly can be bundled together and called dementia that it is worth mentioning these other illnesses.

Mania

Mania and hypomania (meaning a milder degree of mania) are in many ways the opposite of depression. The patient is elated and speeded up, full of wonderful ideas and the energy to carry them out. In severe cases the patient's thoughts come at such a rate that she appears out of touch with her surroundings and acutely confused. Mania is a relatively uncommon disorder, which occurs mainly in people who at other times in their lives have had episodes of depression (*manic-depression* or *bipolar affective disorder*). The patient is her normal self in between episodes, and these periods of good health may last for months or for many years. The onset of mania is usually quite rapid, over days and weeks, so it should not easily be mistaken for dementia.

Paraphrenia

This is also a relatively uncommon condition. It is closely related to the condition of schizophrenia in younger patients, and it is one of the types of *paranoid psychosis*.

The patient, almost always a woman, is usually socially isolated and often made more isolated by deafness. She begins to believe that she is surrounded by persecutors, who get at her and at her property is one or more of a variety of ways. They talk behind her back, spy on her, steal from her house, put in noxious fumes, or interfere with her body.

Such ladies are likely to withdraw socially. Their self-care may decline because they feel that the electricity has been tampered with or their food poisoned. Withdrawal and self-neglect however are the only similarities between paraphrenia and dementia, for otherwise the paranoid patient is fully in possession of her mental powers. Indeed, she may feel that she has to be sharper than usual to keep up with the tricks played by her imaginary persecutors.

Paranoid symptoms are quite common in dementia (p. 181) and in acute confusion (p. 51), but in these cases they are just one part of a much wider syndrome.

Personality disorder

This term is usually applied to a life-long characteristic pattern of attitudes to self, relationships to others and ways of reacting to crises and to the world in general (see also p. 159). A personality type only becomes a personality problem or disorder either when the person herself seeks help because of the consequences of being that type of person, or when it causes problems for others. There have been many descriptions of personality types and personality traits and no exact 'diagnosis' of a particular person's personality type is possible. Each person's make-up is too complicated for that, and so we can only give general descriptions.

Changes with age. As we age the mental changes previously described (p. 36) must affect our personalities. Of course there are many old people who maintain their full personality colour throughout their lives. But for others the tendency towards detachment and less emotional interaction, and the preference for order, regularity and routine which often occurs seem to lead towards a mellowing of the stronger aspects of personality and a move towards a more introverted or more obsessional personality type (p. 161). These are only very general tendencies, but in practice they mean that there are fewer 'psychopaths' among the elderly than among young people. On the other hand, in some people the mental changes of old age bring an exaggeration of certain personality traits, such as hypochondriasis, meanness, dependence, independence, irritability, suspiciousness, obsessionality, so that they become a sort of caricature of their previous selves.

Personality and dementia. As with the other mental changes of old age these changes can all occur in dementia. A dementing person may stay unchanged in personality well into their dementia, may be a quieter version, a 'shadow' of their former selves, or may develop exaggerated or even quite new personality traits. When we notice a change in an old person's personality we need to ask, is this simply a gradual change with old age, is it the beginning of dementia, or is it another psychiatric disorder, a depression or a paraphrenia, which is leading her to behave in uncharacteristic ways? The answer is often difficult because personality is so difficult to define.

The key again lies in the pattern of the change in time. A very rapid change probably indicates illness, either psychiatric or physical; a slow change over months should raise suspicions of dementia; a very slow change indeed over many years is more likely to be simply old age. The other clue is the nature and extent of the change. A slight exaggeration or a mellowing of personality may be a simple ageing. A dramatic change with new personality traits emerging, or ridiculous caricature of the previous personality is much more likely to be due to dementia or to another psychiatric illness.

Indeed, these new developments from the patient's previous personality should not technically be called personality characteristics at all. They have become symptoms and signs of the illness from which the patient is suffering. If the illness is treatable we can hope that she will return to her previous usual personality. The personality changes of dementia are unfortunately not susceptible to treatment, though eventually they are likely to disappear as the illness progresses and the sufferer loses all those characteristic patterns of behaviour that go to make up her personality.

Self-neglect

Of particular interest is that change in personality sometimes known as the *'Diogenes syndrome'* (after the Greek philosopher and teacher of Alexander the Great, who, being a cynic about the values of the world, lived in ostentatious squalor, in a tub). In this syndrome an old person seems to lose all interest in her self-care and care of her house. She lives in appalling squalor, yet seems mentally normal in other ways. Some of these patients also become hoarders, and the condition overlaps with a cleaner, tidier sort of hoarding called *syllogomania* which a few obsessional elderly people become preoccupied with, sometimes to an equally ridiculous extent.

The cause of the gross change in personality in the Diogenes syndrome is not clear. Some patients are probably in the early stages of dementia, some may have suffered a stroke in the frontal region of the brain (see p. 57). But it is also important to rule out the possibility that they have become depressed now or in the past and have neglected themselves because of this, that they have odd paranoid ideas, or that they have suffered from schizophrenia in the past.

Even excluding all these other possibilities there does seem to be a number of elderly people whose personalities change in old age, who *become* eccentric, but do not go on to suffer from dementia. We should realise however that it is much more common for self-neglect and neglect of an old person's house to be signs of the onset of dementia, depression or a physical disability, rather than of this uncommon condition.

Alcohol and drug dependence

These conditions are much commoner among the elderly than most people think. The mental dullness, self-neglect, memory impairment, and periodic episodes of confusion of the addict can easily be mistaken for dementia. The true cause is often missed simply because the right questions are not asked.

Small quantities of alcohol and drugs may lead to quite marked confusion in an old person, so that, although many long-standing alcoholics drink less when they are older, this smaller amount may still be enough to affect the workings of the brain and to cause withdrawal symptoms if it is stopped. There are also 'new' alcoholics, elderly people who for the first time become dependent on alcohol, sometimes out of loneliness, sometimes to deal with anxiety or depression.

Drug dependence particularly on the benzodiazepine drugs such as diazepam and lorazepam is also surprisingly common. It is characterised by dependence on the tablets for day-to-day living, a tendency to increase the dose of the drug and resistance to stopping it so as to avoid withdrawal symptoms.

The patient taking these drugs may feel mentally slowed, with poor concentration and lack of interest, apathy or even depression. These features can seem like dementia. Changes in dose of the drug or stopping it altogether can cause a withdrawal syndrome of acute confusion, often with fits, like delirium tremens. More commonly the patient simply feels very anxious and restless with sleep disturbance.

After a period of days, or a week or so, the withdrawal symptoms fade and she will feel much clearer mentally than before, self-neglect is less, concentration and interest recover. It is then possible to look at any problems such as loneliness or depression which have led to the dependence in the first place.

CONCLUSION

In this chapter I have described a number of conditions which resemble or can be mistaken for dementia. There is endless variety in people's personalities and the illnesses they may suffer. But clear definition of the clinical features and the course of dementia allows us in most cases to make accurate diagnosis, rule out or treat other illnesses and then to concentrate on managing the consequences of the dementia.

3

Who are the dementing and where are they?

HOW MANY SUFFERERS?

Present figures

In Table 1.1 we saw one estimate of the prevalence of moderate and severe dementia among different age groups. We can work out that there are altogether approximately 600 000 moderate and severe dementia sufferers of all ages in Britain in the mid 1980s, of whom about 200 000 are in the 65–74 age group and 400 000 are over 75. So dementia is predominantly a problem for the over-75s, the 'old-old'. A city of 500 000 population would contain about 5000 moderate and severe sufferers, a town of 50 000 would expect 500 and a village of 500 would expect 5 sufferers.

Because of the vagueness of definition at the boundary between dementia and normal old age, it is very difficult to be definite about the figures for milder stages. Some investigators estimate that nearly as many again suffer from mild dementia (which of course will later become more severe). On the other hand some investigators have found a much lower prevalence of all grades of dementia, in some cases as low as half the Newcastle figures. So we can only guess wildly at what is the *actual* number of dementia sufferers in any community. In a way this figure does not matter anyway.

Table 3.1 Population changes in Britain 1901–2001, emphasizing the continuing rise in numbers of those aged over 75, and, even more dramatically, those over 85

Year	Total population within each age group (millions)		
	65–74	75–84	85+
1901	1.3		0.5 (all 75+)
1921	1.9		0.7
1941	3.1		1.2
1961	4.0	1.9	0.3
1981	5.2 (peak)	2.7	0.6
2001	4.7	3.0 (peak)	1.0 (peak not yet reached)
Change from 1901–2001 (millions)	+3.4		+3.5 (75+)
Percentage change	+262%		+700%
Change from 1981–2001 (millions)		+0.3	+0.4
Percentage change		+11%	+66%

What is necessary in order to plan and provide adequate services is to known the *needs* of dementia sufferers — how many people need sitting services, or day hospitals, or long-stay beds. These needs are based on assessment of function, not on diagnosis.

Population changes

There is no dispute about the rapid rise in prevalence of dementia with age. So we can be certain that, whatever the true figures are, they will change considerably over the next 20 years. The proportion of the total population who are in the 65–74 age group is now beginning to fall slowly (Table 3.1), whilst the percentage of these people who are dementing is probably static, so that the actual numbers of dementing people aged 65–74 will be slowly falling. On the other hand, the proportion of the total population who are aged over 75 is rising fast and within that number those over 85 are increasing even faster, so the number of dementia sufferers over 75, and especially over 85, is rising rapidly. The problem of the 'old-old' with dementia is getting worse.

The reasons for these contrary changes in population structure are to be found back in the early years of this century. A 'baby boom' occurred between the 1890s and the beginning of the First World War. Unlike their predecessors most of these babies survived infancy because of gradually improving standards of housing, sanitation and diet. They are now in their late 70s, 80s and 90s. The birth rate has, with ups and downs, been declining ever since that boom. So now, 70 years after the end of the war, the younger age groups, the 'young-old', are declining in numbers, and in 20 years time the older groups will be beginning to decline too.

Sex ratio

Many of those born just before the baby boom, and also many *boys* born during that boom, died in the war and the subsequent influenza epidemic. So the population of 75–100-year-olds contains a very high proportion of women, and an especially high proportion of single women. The fact that men tend anyway to have a shorter lifespan than women means that those women who did marry usually survived, but are now widowed. (The average expectation of life at birth is now about 78 years for a woman but only 73 for a man.)

So, among dementia sufferers there is a large and increasing number of very old people, and, because of the structure of the elderly population, the majority of dementia sufferers are very old women, especially very old women who are widowed or single.

In addition there is evidence that the prevalence rate of ATD (percentage affected at any one time) is greater in older women than in older men, thus increasing further the numbers of very elderly female sufferers. Among younger old people, MID is relatively more common, though still not as common as ATD, and the prevalence rate among men may be greater than among women.

We can immediately see some of the social problems posed by dementia.

WHO IS AVAILABLE TO CARE?

Younger sufferers

The small number of 'pre-senile' dementia sufferers (exact numbers are not known) are likely to have some support at home; they are most likely married with growing up children; they may also have brothers or sisters; they may even have parents! The illness is devastating for these supporters, because it is so unexpected, but at least the supporters exist.

Older women

The older a person is when she develops dementia the less support she is likely to have. An old woman's husband is likely to have pre-deceased her and she may well be living alone. Table 3.2 shows the living conditions of the general population of elderly people at home at different ages. Similar figures for the living conditions of the *dementing* elderly are difficult to obtain because of the difficulty in knowing how many sufferers there are in total (p. 66). Some estimates suggest that 40–50% of sufferers who are at home are living alone, that is, nearly the same figure as for the non-demented

Table 3.2 Where elderly people live (Adapted from Hunt A 1978 The elderly at home. HMSO, London)

6% live in institutions
94% live in private households
Of those in private households, the percentages living alone are as follows:

	Men	Women
65–74	14	34
75–84	20	47
85+	27	50

population. We must at the least assume that many very elderly ladies who are in the early stages of dementia live alone.

This is bad enough in itself, but in addition, if we look for family support for these solitary ladies we are not likely to find much. Children may have moved to other parts of the country or abroad. Children who live nearby will be grown up and working. They are likely to have their own children to look after. Worse still the patient's children may themselves be elderly. So trying to support a dementing parent can cause great disruption to family and social life.

Brothers and sisters, if they are still alive at all, will be elderly themselves and are likely to have their own health problems. If the patient has never married, she may depend on the goodwill of nieces or nephews. So it is now not unusual to find a number of elderly spinster and widowed sisters, some or even all suffering from dementia, being looked after by one or two long-suffering nieces, all that remains of the next generation.

Coping with dementia is a heavy burden for these relatives. On top of this, however, it must be remembered that elderly patients are likely to suffer from a variety of other physical complaints and disabilities as well as dementia.

Older men

For an elderly man with dementia the situation is likely to be different. He is much more likely to have married (because of the relative abundance of women after the First World War) and his wife is much more likely to be alive. Furthermore the traditional role of the woman has been to look after men's needs, and many an older wife may simply be extending what she was already doing in the way of 'care' before her husband became ill. For a traditional husband, on the other hand, looking after a dementing wife is much more difficult. He is being asked to learn completely new skills in housework, cooking and giving personal care so that he can take over from his wife as she becomes less and less capable.

The consequence of these population and social factors is that in practical terms there are three groups of elderly dementing people living at home. First, there is the elderly spinster or widow, living alone with few available supporters. Second, there is the elderly wife or widow living with her husband or children. Third, there is the elderly man usually living with his wife. The needs of these three groups are often quite different, but we will return to that subject when we deal in Chapter 7 with the problems facing families.

WHO SUFFERS?

Who then are the sufferers? The research that is trying to find the causes of dementia has not yet succeeded in identifying any definite causal factors in either ATD or MID, except that both are commoner in old age and that there are genetic factors in ATD.

This means that it does not matter how intelligent or unintelligent a person was previously, or how much or how little she has used her brain, or how stressed or unstressed she is; she is just as likely or unlikely to develop dementia as the next person. No particular occupation carries an increased risk of dementia and as we have seen there has been no definite proof yet that any injury, poison, deficiency or infection is a causal factor in the common types of dementia. So we expect that those who suffer are spread throughout all social classes, all races, all ranges of intelligence, all types of personality.

It is of course likely that different sufferers will try to cope with dementia in differing ways, and have different personal strengths and weaknesses, different family supports and different financial resources to deal with the associated problems. And, as we shall see, the problems presented and the outside help available to deal with these problems will also be very varied, even though the basic process of dementia is the same. So the *experience* of dementia will be unique in each individual case.

WHERE ARE THE SUFFERERS?

Patients at home

Some people find it surprising that any dementia sufferers at all are in their own homes. We can work out very roughly how many are at home by looking first at the percentage of the elderly population who are dementing (Table 1.1), then at the percentage of the elderly population who are in care of any sort (Table 3.2) and finally at the proportion of those in care who suffer from dementia (Table 3.3). We can see that the figures in Table 3.3 are much higher than the figures for the general population in Table 1.1. So there is a concentration of dementing people in institutional care, which is not surprising.

What is more surprising is that when we join all these figures together (remembering that they are approximations and come from rather different sources) we can guess that the great majority of sufferers are *not* in institutions. Surveys have shown that the ratio of dementia sufferers at home to dementia sufferers in institutions may even be as high as 7 to 1.

Community support. So we can see that dementia is largely a problem of community support. Countries and regions differ in how much they rely on institutional care, and how

Table 3.3 The proportion of residents in care who suffer from dementia

Type of care	Estimated proportion who suffer dementia
Psychiatric hospital	45–95% of those aged over 65
Geriatric hospital	45–65% of residents
Acute medical ward	5–15% of those aged over 65
Residential care (Part III or Part IV)	30–70% of residents
Private care	35–75% of residents

The figures are from a number of sources, and show the wide range of estimates which have been made.

much on community care. But there can be few places in the world where the majority, or even a large minority of dementia sufferers are in institutions.

We might imagine that providing some more beds in hospitals or residential homes could help to relieve the burden on the families of the demented. However, if we look at the figures, it is clear that even quite a lot of new residential, nursing home or hospital beds would make little inroad into that proportion of the demented who are at home. Looked at from the opposite direction, however, quite a small relative change in tolerance of the demented by families or communities could put a relatively very large load on the hospital system. Furthermore, since the number of sufferers is constantly increasing, the chances of institutional care 'catching up' with the problem are very slim indeed. Whether we like it or not the 'community' has to learn to care.

Sheltered housing

People who live in sheltered housing form a rather special group. As a general rule, sheltered housing organisations quite reasonably feel that they cannot accept dementing people as residents because of the inevitable decline in self-care which is part of their illness. However, although figures are not available, it is certainly the case that there are many residents living alone in sheltered housing schemes who are at least mildly demented, and some more severely demented residents who are looked after by their spouses.

Psychiatric care

Looking now at those dementing people who are in institutional care of any kind (Table 3.3) we see some major implications for the staff of the various organizations. The figures for psychiatric hospital patients are not too surprising. The elderly in psychiatric hospitals are composed of 3 groups.

'Graduates', presenile and brain damaged patients. The first are those who have grown old in the hospital having been admitted because of schizophrenia or other illness in early or middle life. These go under the somewhat ridiculous name of 'graduates', though their 'graduation' depends on failure

of their treatment and rehabilitation rather than on any success. Included among these graduates will be some patients who have been admitted before the age of 65 because of a 'pre-senile' dementia, and who have survived the years into 'old age', and some patients with brain damage due to head injury, who may expect a normal lifespan with no further worsening of their mental impairment. Included among the larger group of chronic schizophrenics will be some who, separately from their schizophrenia, develop an 'ordinary' dementia in their old age (presumably 5–10% of the total).

'Functional' patients. The second group is of patients admitted after the age of 65 who suffer from psychiatric illnesses such as depression, mania and paranoid psychosis — the so-called 'functional illnesses'. Relatively few of these become longer term hospital patients, partly because many are successfully treated, but also because there are alternative forms of residential care for mildly disabled elderly people which are not available to younger patients. Of course a few of this group develop dementia or are discovered to have it already.

The elderly with dementia. The third group are those who develop dementia in old age and require admission. This is the biggest group and the numbers involved have been expanding steadily over the past 20 years.

Probably less than one in ten elderly dementia sufferers ends their days in a psychiatric hospital. So it is wrong to think of dementia as being the sole responsibility of the psychiatric services. Only those who need specialised psychiatric nursing should be in a psychiatric hospital. These are the patients who as part of their dementia have severe behavioural disorders, emotional disturbances or disinhibition. They are in fact very much a minority of dementia sufferers, and indeed many residents in long-stay psychogeriatric wards probably do not need to be there — their needs are more for physical nursing care or for the type of care that could be given in an EMI home (p. 74).

Geriatric care

Perhaps the figures for dementia in geriatric hospitals are not surprising either. I have already pointed out that many elderly patients with dementia suffer physical illnesses as well as their dementia; and at the later stages of a simple dementia the need for physical care is often the predominant problem. Furthermore, in MID the other consequences of arteriosclerosis (Fig. 1.8) or the strokes which are the essential cause of the dementia can leave the patient with major physical nursing needs.

We should expect, then, that there will be be a high proportion of dementia sufferers in geriatric wards and an especially high concentration of those with multi-infarct dementia. In general, these should be people who are not disturbed and therefore do not need psychiatric care.

General medical wards

In general medical wards the figures are also high. Here there will be some patients who have true acute illnesses and happen also to be dementing. But in many parts of the country shortages of geriatric, psychogeriatric and residential care places lead to misplacement and 'bed-blocking' by patients who are no longer acutely physically ill, or who were admitted with no major medical problem in the first place and who cannot return home (p. 303).

The traditional organization of medical wards, to diagnose and treat complicated medical conditions without much need to investigate the patient's home circumstances or organize elaborate rehabilitiation programmes, tends to work against the needs of the dementing elderly person. She gets stuck and quickly becomes no more than a name on a waiting list for long-term care.

Homes for the elderly mentally infirm (EMI homes)

Homes specifically for the care of dementing people are available only in some areas of the country. Ideally these are for people who do not need specialized nursing care, but who would be a little too disturbed for ordinary residential home care. Where such homes exist they take some of the load away from hospitals, some from ordinary residential care, and some from the community.

Residential and nursing homes

Homes vary greatly in their admission policies with regard to dementia. Most local authority residential homes ('Part III homes' in England and Wales, 'Part IV' in Scotland) wish to accept dementia sufferers only if their impairment is mild and they retain some degree of independence in self-care — dressing, washing, toileting and mobility. They also demand an agreement from the prospective resident that she wishes to enter the home. Theoretically, such an agreement could only be made by a mildly demented person with insight into her dementia, who retained enough reasoning power and understanding to come to an informed rational decision (see Ch. 8).

The figures in Table 3.3 tell a different story. A large proportion of residents in residential homes suffer from dementia. Sometimes the dementia will have begun or progressed after admission, but it is likely that more than half of those admitted to residential care are already dementing.

In homes run by voluntary bodies and private residential and nursing homes the proportion of demented residents will vary depending on their individual policies. Some homes claim to specialize in looking after 'psychogeriatric' patients, some claim that they specifically do not look after this group. But in fact in many such homes the proportion of dementia sufferers is as high as in local authority homes and sometimes even higher.

Statistical problems

The lack of accurate figure in this area emphasizes a general lack of knowledge of what dementia is and how it may be defined. Some homes will have residents who have very poor memories and are beginning not to be able to look after themselves, but who are nevertheless not thought of as 'confused' or 'demented'. There is an implication that 'demented' only refers to dementia with behaviour problems. The term 'psychogeriatric' is used, rather more accurately, to mean the same thing.

The only proper way to assess dementia is by a combination of intellectual and behaviour testing coupled with a view of the course of the illness (see Ch. 9). Only when we have figures based on such assessments will we know exactly where the dementing of our community are.

Even then there is a further problem. For when people go into residential care of any sort they often cross the artifical boundaries of the catchment areas set up by social work departments and health services. These boundaries rarely coincide. So far it has therefore been impossible to define accurately how many people with dementia who originally lived in a particular area are still in their own homes, how many have moved to sheltered housing, how many to residential, nursing home or EMI home care and how many are in hospital either for short-term or longer-term care.

WHO GOES WHERE?

When we look at the proportion of dementing people at home and the figures for different types of care as far as these are available, the question arises: 'Why is one particular sufferer at home, another in residential care, another in hospital?'

Many people in the different sectors of care talk about 'appropriate' patients. We would all like to be able to decide what sort of patient should go to our own sort of care. And for planning purposes it would be helpful to be able to ascertain how much need there is in a particular community for the different sorts of care and from that agree on what to provide: how many home helps, how many sheltered home places, and how many residential care places, how many of the various types of hospital bed. Let us look at what happens in practice. Who goes where, and why?

Severity

The most obvious answer would be that those with mild dementia stay at home, those with moderate dementia go to residential-type care, those with severe dementia are in nursing home or hospital care, perhaps the most severe cases being in geriatric hospitals since the terminal stage of the illness involves the greatest need for physical nursing care.

The facts are very different. If we look at people in these various settings we find all stages of dementia in all settings, mild and severe at home, mild and severe in hospital, etc. Part of the reason for this is that there is a very humanitarian tendency of carers, whoever they are, and wherever they are, to wish for *continuity of care*. They keep on looking after the dementing person long after they are out of their depth, because they know and like the patient, can learn as they go along how to deal with the new problems that arise and know how disturbing a move can be. But we also have to explain why only *some* severely demented people stay at home and, more particularly, why some of the more mildly demented get admitted.

Type of dementia

I have already mentioned that patients with MID are more likely to need specific medical attention, because of strokes and the other problems of arteriosclerosis. For this reason these patients are more likely to be in a medical or geriatric ward. Further, the rather sudden changes in level of impairment and the acute confusional states which may accompany the little strokes of MID are likely to cause minor crises which lead to admission (Table 1.4). The steadier progress of ATD patients and the fact that they are often in excellent physical health throughout most of their decline mean that they are less likely to need specific medical care. Younger patients of any diagnosis tend to be of more interest to neurologists, because of their wider range of alternative diagnoses, such as Huntington's chorea and normal pressure hydrocephalus. This makes investigation more worthwhile and treatment sometimes possible.

But these are only trends. In practice, all types of dementia are found in all types of setting.

Specific problems

The list of 'crises' in Table 1.4 goes a long way towards explaining why it is not only the severely demented who are in care. Any of these crises can occur at any stage of the process of dementia.

Table 3.4 A checklist of the problems which may affect dementia sufferers and their families. The list is not exhaustive!

Problem	Examples
Memory impairment	Forgets appointments, visits etc.
	Forgets to change clothes, wash, toilet
	Forgets to eat, take tablets
	Loses things
Disorientation	Time
	Around house
	Recognizing family or other visitors
Needs physical help	Dressing
	Washing, bathing
	Toileting
	Eating
	Housework
	Mobility
Risks in the home	Falls
	Fire from cigarettes, cooker, heating
	Flooding
	Letting strangers in
	Wandering out
Risks outside	Driving, road sense
	Gets lost
Apathy	Little conversation
	Lack of interest
	Poor self-care
Poor communication	Dysphasia
Repetitiveness	Questions or stories
	Actions
Uncontrolled emotion	Distress
	Anger or aggression
	Demands for attention
Uncontrolled behaviour	Restlessness, day or night
	Vulgar table or toilet habits
	Undressing
	Sexual disinhibition
	Shoplifting
Incontinence	Urine
	Faeces
Emotional reactions	Depression
	Anxiety
	Frustration
	Embarrassment and withdrawal
Other reactions	Suspiciousness
	Hoarding and hiding

Table 3.4 (*cont'd*)

Problem	Examples
Mistaken beliefs	Still at work
	Parents or spouse still alive
Decision-making	Indecisiveness
	Easily influenced
	Refuses help
Burden on family	Disruption of social life
	Distress, guilt, rejection
	Family discord

Indeed, as we shall see in Chapters 5 and 6, the 'crises of behaviour' are more likely to occur *early* in the illness, when the patient still retains the ability to react and interact with others, still has the physical ability and motivation to act, and still has some imperfect insight into what is happening to her. Later, as these abilities are gradually lost, the behaviour problems may dissolve, to be replaced by a passive, withdrawn, insightless contentment. The result is that some mildly demented people are admitted to long-term care because of one of these crises of behaviour, whilst quite severely demented patients may remain at home, as long as they are undisturbed and as long as support for their declining abilities can be gradually increased. The mild cases that *are* admitted may live on in hospital for many years after their disturbed period has passed.

It is not just crises, however, that lead to a demand for admission. The burden caused by any of a long list of problems (Table 3.4) can gradually lead to a situation where relatives feel they can cope no longer.

The next three chapters will explain these problems in more detail, and Chapter 7 will deal with the feelings they evoke in the relatives. If we could develop ways of dealing with these problems we could avoid some premature decisions about long-term care and make 'community care' of the dementing a much more tolerable experience for relatives.

Social factors

Support by families. Perhaps, however, the most important

factors determining whether a dementing person stays at home or goes into care are social. Table 3.2 suggests how this occurs. Dementing patients who live alone with few supporters are the principal users of long-term care. Those who live alone but get regular support are somewhat less likely to need long-term care early in their dementia, whilst those who live with their supporters may survive for much longer periods. Among this last group the crucial factor is whether or not the relatives are willing to continue caring.

It has been shown that where there was a good and strong relationship with the dementing person before the illness began (a good marriage, or a good parent-child relationship), the relative will be inclined to continue through the difficult early stages of dementia and on to the late stages when more physical care is required. Only quite severe problems will make such families want to give up, unless, of course, a deterioration in their own health makes it impossible for them to continue caring. If there has been a bad or weak relationship before, then there will be a general tendency to want to give up when the problems of caring for the dementing person begin to become a burden.

There are variants of these two patterns. Sometimes a bad relationship is nevertheless a strong one; for example, in the case of a couple who are bound together closely but nevertheless argue constantly, or that of a 'martyr' daughter who takes on an impossible load of caring for a domineering parent. Sometimes the relationship can change as the dementia progresses. Occasionally, for example, a difficult, aggressive husband becomes much more placid and likeable when dementing. Rather more frequently, less desirable characteristics emerge as part of the dementia, spoil a previously harmonious relationship, and lead the relatives to the reluctant decision that they must give up caring.

Support for families. So the presence or absence of support and the willingness of the suporters to continue are very important factors. 'Support for the supporters' is also important. Looking after a dementing person is a 24-hour-a-day job and only the most loyal, patient and good-humoured relative can manage this alone. The job of caring is much easier where there is a large family or an extended family (involving different generations, and different degrees of relationship) who can share the time of caring and can support each other.

Such sharing of care is unfortunately the exception rather than the rule in Britain, though more possible in many other countries. Increased social mobility, emigration, small family size, a wish for independence on the part of children and a feeling that a young couple should run their own lives with only their own children to care for, have all led to a decline in mutual family support. And, as already stated (p. 68), it is very often the case that such extensive family support simply cannot exist because the patient is a spinster or a widow with few children.

Our welfare systems have been developed partly to give expert advice and care to people in need of help, but partly also to fill the gaps left by the decline in the ability of families and neighbourhoods to support their disabled relatives or neighbours. It remains a matter of debate whether the existence of such welfare systems encourages supporters to give up supporting earlier than they would otherwise, or at least try to give up, and whether this is 'right' or 'wrong'. But that is not the point here.

For dementia victims and their supporters an either/or dichotomy is unhelpful. It is not a case of the relatives either coping entirely by themselves or giving up entirely. There is a large grey area between these extremes. In this grey area the relatives cope better or worse depending on how supported they feel. If other members of the family, friends or neighbours can give this support, that is well and good; if not, then outside support systems, be they health service, social services, voluntary or private organizations, can fill the gap, working in partnership with the regular supporters and sharing care (p. 289). Most developments in geriatric and psychogeriatric care in the past 20 years have been of this supportive or gap-filling nature.

Buying care. The availability of money can obviously determine to a great extent where a patient can be. It takes money to buy a house with a 'granny flat', allowing an elderly parent to live relatively independently while giving some supervision and support if she begins to dement. Money can buy more 'granny sitting' or nursing care at home than is available from the health or social services in most areas. And it has until recently required considerable amounts of money to afford private care. This situation has been changing with financial support from the Department of Health and Social Security for people who enter a private residential or nursing home and whose capital is below a certain level. It has begun to look as if private care will be accessible only to the very rich and the very poor. The debate continues and these arrangements are likely to change over several years to come.

The use of attendance allowance, mobility allowance and invalid care allowance to buy appropriate care helps to a minor extent in maintaining patients in their own homes. But funding to the same level as that given by the DHSS to support private residential or nursing home care would be needed to make proper community care a possibility for the majority of sufferers and so lessen the burden both on relatives and on institutional care. Experiments in funding community care in this way have been tried in a number of areas.

Availability of services

Money can only buy what is available. A patient's desire to go into care, or the desire of her relatives to give up caring at home, can only lead to admission if a place in an institution is available. It is easy to see that if one form of care is not available in a particular area, then there will be pressure on other services. They will be asked to do a job which they do not consider is theirs to do. They will be asked to take patients who are too fit or too unfit for their service as they see it. The full implications of this are seen in the 'Balance of Care' model (Table 3.5).

In the table we can see that not only is there a range of *types of care* — support at home, day support and residential care — but a range of *providers of this care* — health services, social services, voluntary bodies and private organizations. Whenever help is needed from one of these services then whether or not the service is given or not depends largely on whether it is available. If the service is not available then a load falls on the services on either side or up or down the same column of the table.

If there is no day hospital service for dementia sufferers in

Table 3.5 The balance of care

Type of care	Providers of care (examples) Health service	Social work	Voluntary and private
Home care	Primary care team	Home helps	Sitters
Day care	Day hospital	Day centres	Day centres
Residential care	Long-term hospital	EMI homes Residential homes	Residential homes Nursing homes

a particular area, then other day care services will be taking some of these patients. These other services may justifiably protest that they were set up to do a quite different job — either to be a social club for older people, or, in the case of medical day hospitals, to be a centre of nursing, physio-therapy and occupational therapy for people with specific medical problems (p. 304). Other patients and their supporters will have to struggle on at home with too little support, or causing a load on home care services that they should not have to carry. Some families, with the backing of their general practitioner, solicitor or other advisors will feel they cannot cope and so the patient will be prematurely admitted to care of one sort or another.

To give another example, the widespread absence of EMI homes means that many dementing patients who require supervision and simple basic care are having to be looked after in local authority residential homes which are not staffed or organized to give the necessary supervision and care, in private homes which may or may not have the necessary staffing, or in hospitals where the levels of staffing and training may actually be more than is needed so that money is wasted.

At its simplest, the Balance of Care model shows that we need to have both adequate community supporting services *and* adequate residential care services if the problem of dementia is not going to be one merely of desperate 'gate-keeping', of buck-passing, and of crisis decision-making. It also suggests that, in the meantime, the different services in a particular area should know as much as possible about each other in order to co-ordinate their planning and use of resources, so that the burden of care for patients who need a service that is not yet available is shared equitably.

Admission policies

The situation is made still more complicated by the fact that, to a greater or lesser extent, entry into, or discharge from each 'box' in the balance table is determined by the policies of the 'gate-keepers' and these policies are all too often devised in a vacuum (Table 3.6). The British Geriatric Society and the Royal College of Psychiatrists have drawn up guide-lines to help distinguish between a typical 'geriatric' dementing patient and a 'psychogeriatric' dementing patient, but most other admission policies are drawn up by organiz-ations in isolation, and even the BGS/RCPsych guidelines can easily lead to dispute in a particular case.

What makes some of these admission policies ridiculous is that, whilst they determine admission or non-admission to some extent, the other factors already mentioned are equally or even more important. Thus, a local authority may set up its residential home system with a policy of only accepting residents who have given informed consent to admission. If they stick rigidly to this then the care of dementing people who cannot or will not give this consent falls on the community, on the private sector, or on hospitals — the balance of admission policies determines where a patient ends up. However, if there is a shortage of community supporters or of hospital services in the area, then pressure for admission will outweigh the local rules about admission. Admission policies would be more effective if they were discussed and agreed between the different services (p. 311).

CONCLUSION

We will return to these issues later when discussing the proper organization of help for dementia sufferers in Chapter 10. The importance of looking at these factors now has been to highlight the constraints within which we are all working in trying to care for a dementia sufferer. The next five chap-ters will deal with the actual management of a case of

Table 3.6 Admission policies to care

Organization	Service	Contract	Compulsory powers	Who pays
NHS	Hospital long-stay care	'Treatment contract' often not explicit	Mental Health Act powers rarely used	Free at point of use Pension reduced
Social work departments	Residential care	Signed application	Guardianship rarely used	Client with support from SW
Voluntary organizations	Residential care	Signed application usual	Guardianship rarely used	Client, but DHSS support available
Private organizations	Residential or nursing home care	Application may be made by relative or lawyer	Guardianship rarely used	Client, but DHSS support available

dementia. We will concentrate on how the problems of dementia sufferers and their families arise. We will see that assessing problems and their causes can lead to clear ideas of the best management. But, at the back of our minds, we should be asking whether our plans to help are practically possible. Are the facilities available to manage our patients properly? Will our management materially alter the circumstances of the patient? Or will factors beyond our control determine what happens to her? This may seem a rather pessimistic stance. However, only by being aware of the constraints on our optimism can we see how to improve the outlook for dementia sufferers of the future.

4

The losses of dementia

In this chapter we will look at the most obvious cause of problems in dementia — progressive damage to the brain causing gradual decline in its function. As we have just seen, the *problems* that bring dementing people to medical or other attention are varied and are not all to do with this central process of decline. Some problems arise from the symptoms of disinhibition and reaction described in Chapters 5 and 6, while others are more to do with the family or with social factors. In assessment (Ch. 9) we will see that it is helpful to pin down and list these problems and then to look at what is causing them. So each of the next chapters is about a different *type of cause* of problems in dementia. We will see that one problem, say restlessness (Table 5.2) or depression (Table 6.1) can have a number of causes and will therefore appear in a number of chapters. First, though, we will look at how loss of brain function leads to problems for dementing patients.

Localization of function in the brain

As widespread areas of the brain are progressively damaged in dementia, the functions of those areas decline. We might expect that we could deduce the total effect of a dementia by adding together all these losses of function.

87

Specific functions. As Figure 1.2 shows, there are some parts of the cerebral cortex, such as the visual, auditory, sensory and motor areas, that have very specific functions. Here *electrical activity* in the neurones in very clearly defined tiny areas of the brain can be linked to very specific sensations or actions, for example, light shining on a specific point on the retina, sound of a precise frequency, touch on one area of skin or the tiny movement of a particular muscle. *Damage* by injury, operation or disease to one of these areas, or to the pathways to and from it, can lead to a loss of its specific action or sensation. An *epileptic* discharge in which the electrical change is localized to a tiny bit of one of these areas (called a *focal* fit) would lead to its specific sensation or action occurring out of the blue. These three types of evidence, from measuring electrical activity, from 'lesions' (foci of local damage) and from the effects of focal fits, together with anatomical evidence of connections with other areas, have led to better understanding of what these parts of the brain do. In fact, the diffuse damage of ATD and most other types of dementia tend to spare those areas which have very specific functions, at least until very late in the illness. In MID, however, a localized stroke may damage such areas, or their connections, resulting in a paralysis or a gap in the field of vision, for example.

Wider areas. In other parts of the cortex quite specific functions are carried out by wider areas. Examples include those areas of the temporal and frontal lobes which are concerned respectively with the reception and expression of speech; the secondary sensory areas of the parietal lobe, where we appreciate shape, space and the other aspects of perception that translate sensations into patterns which can be recognized as objects; and the hippocampal region in the temporal lobe which is involved in recent memory. These wider areas are all affected in dementia, and loss of their functions is one of the most obvious aspects of the syndrome. So important is loss of the controlling function carried out by wide areas of the frontal lobes that it is the subject of most of Chapter 5.

General functions. But there are still more subtle types of brain function. Functions like thinking, imagining, storing distant memories, intelligence, emotional responses, personality attributes and social habits are all carried out by making connections all over the brain. So it is impossible to localize any particular area which is specifically involved. It is to these functions that the 'law of mass action' applies; the more damage, the more loss of function, no matter whether that damage is patchy or is worse in one area than another.

In reviewing the losses of dementia, we will see that these very general losses are much more insidious in their development, that they have very general effects on the life of the patient, but that there is very little that can be done to help them. In the case of damage to more specific functional areas assessment of the loss of function is simpler, and it is easier to work out how to help.

Complications in assessing losses

Simply adding up losses does not, unfortunately, describe the whole situation. There are complications.

Patients start their dementia from differing levels of function

A baseline is most important in assessing how much has been lost, but it is difficult to work out in retrospect what someone was like before her dementia began. Even relatives can find it hard to be clear about how she functioned previously, and very careful questioning is required. Putting a specific date on memories of her past can be particularly helpful. 'She used to be able to count her grocery bill quicker than the checkout girl.' 'How long ago was that?'

Losses gradually increase

Dementing patients are rarely in a static position for long; they will usually be getting worse. Assessment of losses should therefore be a continuous process, not once-for-all. And a particular treatment or way of helping will have to be repeatedly reviewed.

Losses appear to vary

As well as this slow decline and the 'step wise' variations in course which may occur in MID (p. 25) there are other reasons why a patient's performance may be different at different times.

Time of day. Many relatives and staff describe a change, somewhere around 4 p.m. or later, after which the patient becomes more disorientated, muddled and restless. There are a number of possible explanations for this phenomenon, including fatigue, a natural search in the evening for familiar surroundings, diurnal variations in hormones, and changes in light. Assessment should take both the morning and evening levels of performance into account.

Fatigue. We can see the effects of mental fatigue on a patient if we ask her to keep doing something such as reading or mental arithmetic for a period. Quite a small 'load' of mental effort fatigues her, she loses concentration and begins to make mistakes. This limits how much assessing and how much activity she can take part in at one session. It also indicates how much 'mental work' she can cope with in her day-to-day life.

Attention. Wandering attention is part of fatigue. As we shall see (p. 124) it is a major problem in dementia. How well the patient performs depends on whether she can attend to the task in hand, or whether there are distractions which take her attention away. A noisy or busy environment will make her perform worse.

Emotional state. When the patient is angry, suspicious, anxious, depressed or unco-operative she is less likely to perform well than when she is in a good mood, confident and inclined to co-operate.

Who is present. Some people have an approach that helps patients to perform. They are probably calmly encouraging and know how to help the patient use her abilities to the best. They sense when her attention is wandering and know to give her a break. Others seem not to be able to do this. The result is that there can be two quite different assessments of the same patient. Sometimes this leads to argument, but in fact both types of information are important. For one tells how good the patient can be in the right circumstances and suggests what we should be aiming for. The other points out how bad she can be and emphasizes problems that can arise. Instead of arguing, the people who are assessing should realize that together they have a full picture of the patient's ability to perform.

Losses mean different things at different stages

As a particular deficit increases, two things may occur which alter its importance. Firstly, its relation to other losses may change, so that the *pattern* of loss changes. For example, insight may change faster than the ability to cope with money. At first the patient's insight will match her deficits and she will realize that she is not managing perfectly. But later the loss of insight is greater than the loss of coping. Although she is now less able to cope with money she thinks that she has little or no problem.

Secondly, different degrees of loss may have different *practical significance*. Thus memory impairment in early dementia may lead to some silly mistakes but no major risk; later on, the greater impairment leads to major risks, of fire, gassing, flooding; later still, if she goes into care, the practical importance of her severe memory loss becomes less again, because there is someone around to care for her and fill in the gaps. As well as reassessing the degree of loss and the pattern of loss it is therefore also important to reassess practical consequences of losses for the person's present life.

Losses interact

Because of the multitude of different types of loss that occur in dementia it is not surprising that losses affect each other in complicated ways. We will see that many different functions must interact to allow a patient to say what time of day it is (p. 97). And if one of these functions, say sense of the passage of time, is lost, all the other interacting functions, such as the ability to name, the ability to remember etc., are rendered useless.

One loss can also make another *appear* worse. Thus if speech difficulties are present either in comprehension or expressing, the patient may seem more disorientated than she actually is, because she cannot understand the question or because she cannot express her answer. Another example of this interaction between losses is the apathetic lady, who has lost her motivation to look after herself as a direct result of the brain damage (p. 113). We might show that her other deficits do not prevent her cooking for herself — she has all the necessary skills — but when we try to get her to cook she does not have the *will* to manage. The two deficits add together and she performs less well than she 'should'.

Disconnection

Very often a particular function seems not to be too badly damaged, but the *connections* between it and other important functions are lost. Thus a patient may be able to understand the words 'sit down' perfectly; she may be able to sit down perfectly; but if she cannot make the connection between the words and the action she will be unable to carry out this simple command, and so will appear extremely confused (or obstinate). Disconnection is extremely common in dementia. It interferes with many functions and it is very difficult to overcome. We will see several other examples later in this chapter.

Assessing and management

As we now examine some of the losses of dementia in detail we will see some general principles of assessment and management emerging.

Management often depends on looking at a loss in two different ways. The first is 'What can the patient not do?' But perhaps more important is the second question, 'What can she still do?' Assessment needs to be able to answer both questions. And the answers to the two questions will suggest different approaches to treatment. We can try to *fill the gap* of what is missing by external aids. Or we can try to ensure that the patient is using what she has left to the full — we can *stimulate* and encourage functioning. In a few cases *retraining* can actually extend the amount of remaining function and so reduce the gap. We will see how these different approaches suit the various losses to a greater or lesser extent.

Firstly, we will consider impairment in the ability of the brain to take in information, for everything that we do depends on our understanding of the world about us. Then we will look at failures in the storage of information. Next we will examine general losses in the processing abilities of the brain, and finally expression and action. This is the best sequence to follow, for each of these types of loss interferes with the next, and there is less interaction back along the list. Thus a difficulty in understanding speech affects the patient's ability to express speech (p. 94). But a difficulty in expressing speech will not affect her ability to understand others.

RECEIVING INFORMATION

Perception

Agnosia

Many perceptual difficulties can arise from progressive damage to the function of the parietal lobes, which is common in ATD. For example the functions of feeling or seeing the shape of something, appreciating the position of an object in space, distinguishing right from left and recognizing faces all involve parietal areas. These are part of the process of perceiving what objects are.

The practical effects of such losses, which mostly go under the name of *agnosia*, are numerous. If common objects are not perceived properly they may be used for the wrong purpose or become useless. Agnosia goes some way to explaining why a dementing lady puts the milk in the sugar bowl or does even more risky things, like putting her underclothes under the grill, although poor attention, dyspraxia (see p. 118), perseveration (p. 128) and poor connections in her thinking may also be involved. Impaired ability to see things in space may explain why she misses her chair, although poor mobility may also play a part. Poor localization of bodily sensation creates difficulties in complaining about or diagnosing physical illnesses. Agnosia puts a great barrier between a patient and the outside world. It can lead to dangers in the home and limits her ability to use everyday objects, or indeed do anything to care for herself.

Recognition

An added problem is that the sense of *familiarity* of an object, place or person may be lost. In focal epilepsy of the temporal lobe a patient may have the experience of *déjà vu* (the feeling that an unfamiliar object has in fact been seen before) or *jamais vu* (that a familiar object has never been seen before). We can therefore guess that this type of recognition is a function of the temporal lobes. In dementia this function is gradually lost. The result is that even though the patient perceives her room as *a* room, and can understand what the objects in it are, yet she does not recognize them as *her* room and *her* objects. The consequences of this jamais vu or strangeness can be that she wants to 'go home' from her own house; or that she thinks people are bringing in strange furniture or objects; or that she wishes to put the strange man, who is actually her husband, out of the house.

Perception of speech

The recognition of words from out of the millions of sensations of sound that go to the auditory cortex is a function mainly of the temporal lobes. Damage here leads to a lack of understanding of what is heard, called *receptive dysphasia*. Dysphasia means difficulty with speech. Reading ability resides in the parietal lobe and damage here can lead to *dyslexia*.

These difficulties in recognizing words in speech or writing apply not only to what *we* say or write to the patient. They also affect her own words. She does not know whether she has said or written sense or not, and so may produce rubbish words without apparent concern. So any attempt to communicate to her or by her becomes difficult.

Understanding

At a 'higher', more general level, the dementing patient's capacity to *grasp* the situation and *understand* what is going on, to get *meaning* out of it, declines. Consequently, she may misinterpret her situation or be bewildered by it. Again, she will have difficulty in realizing the problem and so may appear unconcerned. She understands little but acts as if she understood the situation fully.

These problems of general grasp usually involve loss of the

connections between perception and logical reasoning. A patient may, for example, see that it is dark outside, and be able to say so, and yet not connect that accurate perception logically, so she says that it is the middle of a lovely day. She may see and understand the meaning of the word 'Toilet' on a notice, but walk past it because she does not connect it to the feeling that she needs the toilet now. Her good perception has been useless.

Assessment of perceptual losses

There are a number of 'parietal lobe tests' which identify agnosias. For example deficits in this area can be shown by difficulties in recognizing by touch alone objects placed in the hand, and by difficulties in copying shapes accurately without missing bits out or distorting them. Receptive dysphasia is most easily tested by checking if the patient can follow instructions of an increasingly complicated nature, starting with, say, 'Stick out your tongue', going on to 'Touch your nose with your left little finger'. It is important also to test reading ability.

Management of receptive losses

Most ways of trying to help any disabled person demand their understanding of what is happening — instructions, physical aids, activities. It is very difficult therefore to help someone who has a problem in perception or understanding. If she is not aware that there is a problem, as is so often the case, things are even worse, for she will not see the need for help.

Simplifying. The first principle is to lighten the load of information. We should give very simple instructions, use simple aids and activities, and avoid confusing matters by long explanations which may merely be misinterpreted. The patient also needs encouragement to simplify *her* speech and actions. We should intervene and try to pin her down to simple answers, or to doing one action at a time. For she will tend to ramble on, not realizing that her speech and actions are not making sense.

Getting round the problem. A second approach is to avoid the problem and try to get information across by another route. Thus if reading is difficult picture messages, or 'charades' may help, though unfortunately much of our thinking, even about pictures is done in words. If recognizing objects or places is a problem then a label or notice ('Toilet') can sometimes help. The speech therapist may have particular ways of getting round problems of reception of speech. But there will be great difficulty in giving any form of help when it is the more general aspects of understanding that are impaired. We are likely to end up having to do things for the patient, rather than help overcome the problem.

Attention and concentration

Attention is the ability to focus one's mind and consciousness on a particular object, task or thought (see p. 124). Concentration is the ability to sustain attention over a period of time. Even if we can gain the patient's attention, and even if she can perceive what we say, she may not be able to keep concentrating long enough to take in all the information we give. Poor concentration is very common in dementia and it causes enormous problems not only in receiving information but in action as well. Relatives frequently complain that they could cope much better if only the patient could sustain some activity. She sits down with the paper and attends at first, but quickly loses concentration and wants to do something else. She starts to cook a meal and drifts off in the middle, leaving a saucepan to burn dry.

This inability to settle at anything inevitably leads on to the problem of restlessness. But most of all it interferes with our attempts to help. Any reorientation or retraining programme may founder because the patient's concentration cannot be maintained. She simply gets up and walks off. This can make group activities in particular rather disorganized affairs. In severe dementia the ability to attend is lost completely so that engagement in any activity is impossible and little in the outside world 'gets through' to the patient.

A repeated and active effort by family or staff to gain the patient's attention can overcome the problem to some extent, but she may then become easily fatigued or, feeling the pressure on her, collapse in emotion (p. 135). Games and other activities in which she can feel involved could improve concentration. It might even be possible to devise simple variants of the video games which engross younger people and so extend concentration in time, but it remains to be seen how much of this improvement would generalize to other activities.

Orientation

Orientation is not a simple function. There is no 'orientation centre' in the brain. Our knowledge of where we are in time, place and person depends on the combination of a number of functions.

In order to know what time of day it is, we need an inner sense of the passage of time and continuity; we need a recent memory of what has already happened today or when we last looked at the time; we need a longer-term memory of what usually happens at this time of day; we need to have evidence from our senses, about the light, about what other people are doing; we need to be able to connect all this logically to a particular time. Alternatively we need to be able to read a watch or clock and understand the significance of what we have read. Or we must be able to recall what time we were told it was by someone else. To know the day, week, month or year requires even more memory function. And all require the ability to grasp the question being asked, process it properly and express the answer in words either to ourselves in thought or to others in speech. Similar skills, together with a sense of space and the ability to recognize objects, places and faces, are required for orientation in place and person.

Verbal and behavioural orientation. We can describe two general types of orientation, *verbal* orientation and *behavioural* orientation, depending on whether the ability to speak is involved. Many patients cannot *say* where they are, or cannot use words to *think* where they are, but are nevertheless orientated to the geography of their home or ward. Many cannot tell the time, but can still do roughly the right things at the right time of day. This is behavioural orientation based on using the senses, both outer and inner, as opposed to verbal orientation. Other patients can *say* what the time is, or where they are, but act as if they were disorientated because they cannot connect their verbal knowledge to practical action.

Testing orientation. The questions which test orientation are 'What time is it, what day, what month, what year?' 'Where are you, what is this place?' and 'Who are these people around you?' (not 'Who are you?' which is a question of identity). As with all tests of mental function, orientation tets need careful interpretation to work out which actual functions are impaired. And another single serious defect, for example, in sight or speech, can make someone appear much more disorientated than they actually are.

Importance of orientation. Orientation questions, properly interpreted, can thus be useful as part of a very general check of brain damage. It is important, though, to assess also the practical importance of orientation for the patient. A person at home needs a general sense of time of day, and usually needs to know what day it is. Months and years are less important. In a residential home, knowing mealtimes is useful but other orientation in time is not essential. Orientation in space is vital in one's own home. In a residential home knowing the name of the home is not important, but knowing the way to the toilet and the bedroom is vital. Orientation in person can prevent a lady at home being exploited by bogus workmen. In care it is merely reassuring to know who people are.

Helping orientation depends partly on helping each of the skills involved in this complex process. But there are some general ways of helping, including reality orientation programmes and orientation aids.

Reality Orientation (RO)

This technique was first used in the USA in the 1950s, in the back wards of big mental hospitals, where elderly long-stay residents (many not suffering from dementia at all) tended to have withdrawn and got out of touch with everyday life. The results later encouraged the use of RO for dementia sufferers.

Suitable patients. Basically, the technique consists of presenting the facts of orientation repeatedly to patients,

usually in a group, with positive reinforcement and encouragement. We would not expect such a technique to reverse
the process of dementia, and, if a patient has some specific
deficit in speech or spatial sense etc., a general group technique like this is unlikely to be helpful. Furthermore, it is
unlikely that patients who are severely demented would be
in touch enough to be helped. On the other hand, RO is
likely to help patients who are withdrawn and are therefore
not using their remaining faculties to the full, and those who
lack confidence.

Technique. A group of dementia sufferers, no more than
six if possible, sits in a group. Communication is difficult for
bigger numbers and distractibility becomes a major problem.
Special help should be available for those who are partially
deaf, so that they can hear the rest of the group, and for the
partially sighted. It is important to focus the attention of the
group, by repeated reminders of the subject and by the use
of a reality orientation board, which has the questions of
orientation on it. The questions on the board should be
answered during the session. The patients are thus actively
involved in putting on the board the day, date etc., the place,
the weather, items of news or events happening in their lives
or in the world at large.

The person in charge adopts an encouraging attitude, not
showing up a patient's disorientation but helping her work
out the facts, encouraging her to use her senses to find the
answers to the orientation questions, and praising her when
she is even moderately successful. The patients should also
be encouraged to help each other in working out the
answers. The leader does not criticize or blame patients for
failure. What is said in later sections (p. 104ff) about the need
for a slow pace, calm, simplicity, repetition, cueing and
forced choice to help recall memories are all vital if RO is to
be effective.

Effects. The question whether RO like this is effective
remains open. There is some evidence that it is partly effective over short periods. What is certain is that the technique
has a generally stimulating effect on patients and can improve
morale and interest among staff. So it should not be
dismissed.

24-hour orientation

Possibly more important than the specific technique of reality orientation groups is the fact that from it has grown the idea of carrying on RO techniques throughout the day. It is unlikely after all that patients will remember the facts of orientation learnt in a 'classroom'. In fact, the techniques used in '24-hour orientation' are really designed to help a number of the different deficits that add up to disorientation, and so will be discussed in other sections as well.

Family and staff are asked to remind the patient repeatedly of orientation, and to correct disorientation. This should be done, not in a disapproving way, and not by simply telling her the right answers. She can be asked to use her senses to work out where the place is, reminding her of familiar objects or people 'Who are those people there?' 'Nurses.' 'So where are we now?' 'A hospital.' She can be asked to use her memory to work out the time 'Have you had your lunch yet?' 'Yes.' 'So what time of day will it be now?' 'Afternoon.' As with RO a positively encouraging approach works best. This enables her to use her abilities to the full and it may even be that with training she will improve her ability to work out where she is or what time it is. The verbal element (knowing the name of the place, for example) is always less important than the *behavioural* (finding her way around); and gaining her *active participation* (helping her find her way to the toilet by herself) teaches better than simply giving information ('The toilet is the third door on the right').

Orientation aids

External aids to orientation are also important. Clear, simple labelling of rooms or objects can help, but once again the active participation of the patient in learning to use aids is vital. It is not helpful just to put a 'Toilet' sign up. The patient should be directed to it, asked to read it and then reminded of the association between going to the sign, reading it and finding the toilet. The placing of signs is important. They should be at eye level, and they should stand out well from the background, so that there are no distractions.

The orientating attitude

But encouraging orientation depends most of all on the attitudes of family or staff. If they take the attitude that a dementing person is bound to be disorientated and therefore cannot be expected to tell the time or find her way around, then they will tend to take over and allow her to give up working out where she is. The result is that she will withdraw from day-to-day reality. If they assume that 'dwelling in the past' is normal in dementia, they will let her talk of long dead people as still alive, or talk of going to work without helping her correct her mistakes. If they take a critical view they may argue with her over orientation.

The 'orientating' attitude is one which gently reminds of present reality, and gently corrects mistaken ideas. If she loses her way, we help *her* to find it again. If she thinks she should be at work, we help *her* remember how long it is since her retiral. She is actively involved in working these things out, and so should not feel criticized. This attitude involves hard work, time, repetition and patience. It will not succeed in completely orientating the disorientated, or correcting all mistaken beliefs. But it can help the patient's confidence in using her own senses. It can make her feel less detached and improve the relationship between family and patient or staff and patient.

This is not true in all cases. A few sufferers are upset or irritated by attempts to help them orientate and it is most important that these techniques should be used sensitively and with respect.

STORING INFORMATION

Memory

There are several stages involved in memory. If we come across a new word, say 'Alzheimer', we must first be able to hold it in *attention* and *perceive* it properly. Then we *register* it in a store, 'coded' in a way that will help its recall. Thus to register it better we must make links with dementia — it must have some *meaning*. If there is some *emotional* connection with the word (a relative suffers from ATD) or it is otherwise important (for an exam, for example) that will encourage registration. And we can further improve our chances of recalling the word if we note that it begins with 'A', sounds German and is part of 'ATD' — using mnemonics. When stored there may be a *time or place* coding as well as coding by meaning ('I heard the word *then* and *there*'). So we can place memories in sequence. The store will gradually decay (we *forget* the memory) and we need *reinforcement* of the memory from time to time if it is to persist. Finally, we need to be able to *recall* it, using its coding, so that when we think of types of dementia, or other associated ideas or feelings, the word Alzheimer is 'waiting' ready for use.

Short- and long-term memory

The very short-term retention which amounts to keeping a memory in attention for a few seconds is called *short-term or primary memory*. There is a limit to the number of items that we can normally keep in this memory store; this can be checked easily by testing the number of digits that we can keep in mind long enough to repeat back immediately (the *'digit span'* test). Most people can manage no more than the seven figures of a telephone number (unless they can 'code' a number into chunks, as in 10661939452468). Retention for any longer than seconds involves a more elaborate mechanism called *recent memory*, and retention from months or years ago is called *remote memory*. Many psychologists make no distinction between recent and remote memory calling it all *long-term memory* or *secondary memory*. So long-term memory may involve anything from remembering what we had for breakfast (recent) or events from our school days (remote). Most items of memory enter the long-term store from the short-term store. If we do not have a special reason for storing the word 'Alzheimer' and so do not encode or rehearse it, it will disappear from memory after a few seconds of first reading it. Seeing it or hearing it several times and realizing its importance helps get it stored in the longer-term memory.

Types of memory

There are many different things that we have to remember.

Most is known about memory for words and numbers. But there is also memory for other information from the senses, including visual memory for shapes, objects and people, memory for nonverbal sounds such as music, and memory for smells, tastes and bodily sensations; *geographical* memory, which is the ability to remember one's way around by having a mental map of an area; and there is a sort of muscular memory or memory for actions or gestures that we use (*procedural* memory).

Memory in dementia

Since memory involves attention, perception, thinking and imagining (to work out codes), sense of time and place and the ability to store enormous quantities of information and to recover it when needed, we can guess that a good memory requires that many areas of the brain and their interconnections are working well. There is a problem in all aspects of memory function in dementing patients. Arguments among psychologists about which aspect is *most* affected apply to the milder stages. In the most severely demented people we must assume that there is little or no registration, storage or recall of any type of memory.

Temporal lobe structures are particularly important in recent memory and the temporal lobe is damaged in most, if not all, dementing people. Indeed, in ATD there is quite selective damage to the hippocampus and surrounding structures. This is the area which is also damaged in Korsakoff's syndrome (p. 55), in which recent memory becomes very severely impaired. But the more widespread damage in dementia means a more general destruction of memory functions.

Short-term memory. Unlike patients with Korsakoff's syndrome, dementia sufferers show an impairment of short-term memory. This may be connected with their difficulty in attending. The result is that a dementing person will be able to hold fewer items in the short-term store than a normal person. So she may be unable to keep a telephone number in mind while she dials it, or keep the shopkeeper's total bill in mind while looking in her purse, or keep the amounts of money she is counting in mind as she counts it, or keep anything more than a simple instruction in mind whilst carrying it out (such as 'go through that door and turn left'). The widespread and disastrous effects on every aspect of life that follow this loss can be easily imagined.

We cannot trust the short-term store of a dementing person. We should expect the patient to be able to cope with only one or two bits of information at a time. We should split information into small components, or else try to use other types of memory if more complex information has to be remembered.

Long-term memory. But longer-term memory, both recent and remote, is impaired as well. Part of the recent memory problem follows naturally from the short-term problem. For if a patient cannot hold a memory in the short-term store she will not be able to register it in the long-term store. Remote memories from before the dementia began are in the store already and so do not suffer because of the short-term memory problem. But these stored remote memories decline too and are forgotten. Gradually the patient remembers less and less of their earlier life, leaving only islands of very firmly fixed memories, and eventually nothing at all.

In early stages of dementia the greatest defects may be in coding and retrieval. The patient has difficulty in putting a *meaning* on the memory by associating it with other things so as to store it in a particular mental 'compartment'. She has difficulty associating the word Alzheimer with the compartment labelled 'dementia' and linking it with other ways of remembering such as 'begins with A', 'German name' 'ATD'. And, even if it is stored, there is difficulty using these associations to retrieve the memory. But in addition to these problems it is likely that the actual store of memories decays, i.e. the word Alzheimer cannot be recalled because it has been lost from the store. And recognition must be impaired — she cannot recognize the word as one she has seen before even though it has been properly stored (p. 93).

Management

Self-help. How can we help these problems? Retraining memory to improve it might seem attractive, but there is no evidence that this works. However, the patient may be able to find ways of making more effective use of her existing memory. The difficulty of registering memory may be helped if she rehearses the memory over and over again, and by mnemonics (coding by initials, rhymes or other associations). The problem of storing can be overcome if she writes things down, so that the memories do not have to be stored mentally to the same extent. She will be able to learn these techniques up to a point. However we should always assess how far she can go. The patient who ends up rehearsing a name but cannot remember its significance, or who remembers a mnemonic but cannot remember what it is for ('I had to remember something beginning with N') or has a pile of scraps of paper with reminders which she cannot understand, will simply be anxious or frustrated.

Outside help. We can encourage better use of the patient's memory by outside help. Registration of a word or fact can be helped by offering links and mnemonics to help remind her of its meaning. Storage is helped if the information is repeated from time to time. Recall can be helped by two useful methods. One is called *cueing* and involves giving a hint of the answer or part of the answer, or reminding the patient of a mnemonic. Some mildly demented people can use cues very well. ('What you had to remember was about your money.') The other method is *forced choice*. A list of possible answers is given and the patient is asked to pick out the correct one. If recognition is retained better than 'free' recall, then this method can be particularly helpful. We should not say, 'Who visited you?' but 'Was it the nurse, or the doctor, or your sister who visited?'. Loss of time sequence of memories is more difficult to deal with. The correct sequence may have to be put in by family or staff ('That happened a long time ago, didn't it?' 'That was before you retired.') so that old and new memories are correctly distinguished.

Using the types of memory. Another way to help memory is to use the different types of memory more extensively. If verbal memory is most affected, then visual presentation may be more effective: not 'I'm leaving your money in the drawer,' but 'Look, here's your money, I'm leaving it in that drawer there.' Better still may be memory through action: 'Come, we'll put the money in the drawer.' 'Do you remember where you put the money? Show me where it is.' Best of all is to use as many types of memory as possible for the same thing.

In *reminiscence work*, where the idea is to stimulate old memories, talking over old times is not enough. Pictures, music, dancing, actions (using an old style iron, actions used at work) and even tastes or smells can often bring a much richer recall that is both satisfying to the patient and informative to others.

Lightening the load. Where these techniques do not work, or have limited effect, we may have to lighten the load on the patient's memory. The most obvious way to do this is to *simplify* the information that the patient needs to remember, and advise her against trying to remember too much ('There are only two things you need to remember today'.).

The other way is to provide an *'external store'*. I have already described how she may learn to do this for herself by making notes or 'memoranda'. More often the store has to be provided by others. Thus if she has to remember that Tuesday is pension day, the memory can be stored on a notice board, or in a relative's memory. She then finds out by looking at the board (assuming that she has a way of knowing which day is Tuesday and can find the board!) or the relative can ring up to remind her. She will need a lot of encouragement to use the aids that we provide ('Always look at the board'). Many mildly demented people admit that they have given up using their own memory and instead use their spouse or children as a memory store.

The future. Few people over the age of 30 have learnt to use computers early in life when very fixed memories can be formed. New learning (p. 109) is extremely difficult for dementia sufferers. This means that it will be some decades before significant numbers of elderly sufferers will be familiar enough with computer techniques to make much use of their artificial memories. If electronic aids to memory are to be devised they will have to be in a form that the patient can cope with. Even a digital watch or a pocket calculator is likely to be, and remain, a mystery to the majority of sufferers who did not learn their use as children or young adults. And messages that appear on a TV screen are more likely to bewilder and frighten a dementing person than to help.

However, simple memory aids can be developed. The most useful is a clock or watch which can give a spoken or printed reminder of something the patient has to do at a particular time. This can help pill taking, getting up in the morning, eating a meal that has been left. But the patient has to be able to understand the messages and will need considerable training in using such aids.

Reminiscence

Reminiscence is a normal part of old age. It is normal for an older person to look back over her life, review its ups and downs, perhaps dwelling especially on the good things, and try to put it all in perspective. This is healthy and can be very enjoyable. For many the *sharing* of memories is stimulating. From this has arisen a variety of activities ranging from local history groups to 'reminiscence theatre', from old time song and dance sessions to slide shows of old scenes.

Reminiscence like this is recreational. But it may also be therapeutic. For older people may have unfinished business from the past — regret, bitterness, sadness, anger, guilt and disappointment — which still affects their lives. There may be a relative who has never been forgiven, some distressing event that has never been talked about in the family, wishes and hopes that have never been fulfilled. Discussing these things can help the process of putting the past in perspective.

In both recreational and therapeutic reminiscence, sensitivity is needed. For one person's past joy is another's disappointment, and we can be surprised at the distress caused by old memories. Some people are actually stuck with their memories and do not wish to change. They have bad memories but have no wish to forgive or forget them. They do not use reminiscence positively but dwell on these bad memories. Others avoid any bad memory and look at the past through rose-tinted spectacles.

Reminiscence in dementia. For dementing people this review of remote memories can be useful, particularly as a stimulating recreation. In the absence of new recent memories being laid down the dementing person has only her remote memory to fall back on. And with the uncertainties and confusion of her present life those old memories can be an important solid support. They are in a way the only real evidence she has of her identity as a person.

So her *confidence* can be improved by reminiscing. And the amount of material that comes from her store of memories can be surprising. Using the different types of memory — old tunes, pictures, going to old haunts, using scrapbooks, handling old household implements, going to a local museum, even cooking — can help her get access to that store in a way that her day to day life does not. The delight of recognition and the even greater delight of being able to *explain* something to a younger person is a great help. Here too, emotional reactions may vary, however, for some old memories can be upsetting.

It is best if reminiscence is combined with a reality orientation approach (p. 101). We should not expect dementing people to do much therapeutic work on the past; they are unlikely to be able to change their attitudes to people or events of the past, to come to terms, to reconcile or otherwise put the past in emotional perspective. But we can try to use memories to help the patient understand the passage of time — that those things happened years ago, that things are different now, that those relatives are now dead and that another generation has come along, that it is 20 years since retirement etc. Once again, sensitivity is needed. This reality can be very shocking. Finding out, as if for the first time, that one's husband is dead, or that one is no longer at work, is distressing. If we do introduce reality, we must be prepared to cope with these reactions. We must learn to remind gently and not force the truth on to the patient.

Reminiscence work with the dementing is, however, generally very rewarding. The stimulation of memory, the release of positive emotions and the confidence gained from remembering at all seem to increase the patient's interest and altertness at least temporarily. Even more than with reality orientation, reminiscence helps family and staff to see the real person, their background, achievements and personality, in a way that improves *their* interest and respect. It is engaging for both.

New learning

Dementing patients have to cope with many new situations both due to the ordinary changes of life and as a consequence of their dementia. They have to cope with new home situations, new people, new places and new routines. Unfortunately, they have great difficulty in new learning. Learning is another very general function of the brain and requires the making of multiple complicated connections. It overlaps, of course, with memory function but requires other abilities as well.

For example, if a lady needs to learn to use a new cooker, she must be able to manipulate the controls, remember that it is new, remember what she has been told about it, and think out how it works. As well as having specific deficits in these areas, she will show a general loss of ability to learn new actions. We should not expect her to do well.

It is a wise, general rule, therefore, to keep new learning to the minimum. If it is vital for her to learn something new then the task should be simplified, the instructions should be repeated often and she should be actively involved. Like all other deficits, it is not the case that the ability to learn is lost absolutely; it is slowed down and more difficult. Repeated reinforcement, reminders, praise and rehearsal will be necessary to ensure any significant amount of new learning. It is no wonder that dementing people avoid new experiences and fall back on old learning. Indeed, before thinking of teaching her something new, we should ask ourselves whether her old way of doing things could not still be useful. Thus, if she was not safe with the gas, could the gas cooker not be made safer for her, rather than her having to learn new skills with an apparently safer electric cooker?

Old learning

Much of what we do is done by routine. We learn slowly over many years how to go to the toilet, to feed, to cook, to shop, to do our work, to follow social customs, to communicate with others, to relate to others, to have sexual relationships, to pursue interests and activities. Thereafter all these activities have an element of routine about them. Our brains have a vast store of this learned behaviour ready for our day to day needs. Again there is no special learning *area* in the brain; the store involves connections between widespread areas. So stored learning becomes damaged in dementia. The result is that all these habits decline, so that the patient is less and less able to perform them according to her routine.

Let us take social habits as an example. Normally we respond to others in routine ways. If someone comes up and smiles, we look at them and smile back, we exchange pleasantries, we do things by gesture and facial expression which encourage them to speak. All these actions were learnt years ago. If, however, we were to lose the ability to behave in these ways we would seem unresponsive and would not encourage the other people to respond to us. They would not be inclined to go on with the conversation and might even think that we were being rude.

Similar problems can affect all our routine and not so routine activities. Indeed, it is the less routine that will disappear first. A lady may seem to be able to cook, preparing the same one or two dishes every day. It is only when she tries to cook a dish that she has occasionally done in the past that the loss of learned habits becomes obvious. Loss of old learning can thus hide behind routines. In general Ribot's law (p. 7) applies — things learnt earliest in life disappear last. So social habits tend to decline before personal care, cooking skill before eating skill. But this is only a very general rule.

Can patients be retrained? The answer is probably that *re*training the patient in abilities that have *recently* declined is more likely to work than trying to train her in completely new activities. It is generally easier, for example, for a dementing person to relearn old routines in her own house than to learn a few simple new routines in a new house. For the old learnt patterns are not lost altogether at first. They are merely less accessible, though eventually they will disappear. Unfortunately some professional staff seem more willing to be involved with assessing deficits than to spend their time and patience helping dementia sufferers relearn some of their old habits. Time spent in practising simple but important skills such as cooking, dressing, or using money can be invaluable.

PROCESSING INFORMATION — GENERAL LOSSES

Speed

All older people are slower mentally than they were in their younger days (p. 37), but dementing people slow even more. This slowing affects every aspect of mental activity — reception, storage, central processing and expression — and it progressively worsens.

Anyone who has to deal with a dementing patient must also slow down, for there is no way of remedying the loss of speed. That means talking slowly, moving slowly, allowing her time to think. It means that, given enough time, she may slowly dress and wash herself, slowly learn her way around a new house, slowly remember that her husband has died.

Intelligence and problem-solving

Intelligence is a mixture of abilities. It is mostly concerned with the ability to solve problems but may best be defined as 'what is measured by intelligence tests'. As we age, our scores in intelligence tests may fall, but some of this is due to the normal slowing and cautiousness of old age (p. 37). In dementia there is a definite progressive decline in intelligence, particularly where the tests involve solving new types of problems rather than going over well learnt material. This explains a great deal about the behaviour of dementing patients. They do not handle new problems well, and try to avoid them, whilst they cling to their remaining old knowledge repetitively and to the boredom of others.

Thinking and imagining

Most thinking involves words and so declines as speech deteriorates in dementia. Much of our thinking is also to do with problem solving — 'using' our intelligence — but there is a more abstract form of thought which involves letting ideas float freely through our minds, and which includes imagination and imagery, fantasy and day-dreaming. Although this is not directly to do with solving problems it forms the background of much of what we do. What we think of people, our attitudes to various courses of action, our wishes and desires are all dealt with by this sort of thinking. Both thinking and imagining involve *abstraction*, the ability to move away from the particular object or situation to general concepts and ideas. And there is often an *emotional* content in our thinking.

Like all general functions of the brain thinking of either sort requires multiple and widespread connections; there is no specific 'problem solving' or 'imagining' centre in the brain. And having *new* thoughts must involve the ability to make new connections.

All these abilities decline in dementia. So dementing people imagine less, cannot think abstractly as well as they used to, and do not make new connections, or make mistaken ones (p. 147). In the absence of new thinking the patient has to fall back on the remnants of old thoughts. So her mind will be relatively empty apart from repetitive stereotyped thoughts and platitudes which she cannot develop.

Emotions

The experience and expression of emotion are complex. A person's emotional state changes depending on what she sees or hears, what she is thinking or imagining, what relationship she has with the people or things around about her. And there is a steady state of emotion, the 'mood' that we are in. The *expression* of emotion (see also below p. 137) involves co-ordination of many of the body's mechanisms, for smiling, laughing, crying, blushing, angry gestures, frightened or anxious reactions, sexual expression. Both the content and the tone of what we say are involved. The *experience* of emotion is partly the experience of going through these expressive actions, and partly a more internal, abstract experience. Widespread areas of the brain, especially in the temporal lobes and the centre of the cerebral hemisphere, are involved in emotion, so it is no wonder that all aspects of emotion may be damaged or disconnected in dementia.

Emotions in dementia

Poverty. The principal result is a gradual decline in emotions, called poverty of emotion. The patient simply does not feel or express so much emotionally. The expected ups and downs in mood do not happen. The eventual result is a patient who shows no emotion at all and is totally bland. Since emotional reactions are part of one's personality this decline contributes to the loss of personality often described in dementia. It tends to make her less interesting to others; she is less colourful. And it affects her motivation, so that she is less moved to action by her emotions. But it also allows her not to feel the full horror of her situation.

Disconnections. Disconnection between emotions and their causes and disconnection from their expression are also common. For example, a patient may talk about a distressing personal subject without apparent emotion. Another may say that she feels distressed but does not express the feeling in her face and gestures. Another may do the opposite and be, for example, in tears without seeming to feel distressed. These phenomena of lack of emotion and loss of emotional connections contrast with the loss of control of emotion described in Chapter 5.

Management. There is no way of putting back the lost emotions. We simply have to learn to live with a patient who does not respond emotionally. However there are also some people who *appear* to have become dull and emotionless when in fact they have simply become withdrawn (p. 181). These patients can 'come out of their shell' with the right stimulation. It is also important to distinguish poverty of emotion from depression, either as a reaction to dementia (Table 6.1) or as part of a depressive illness; to distinguish it from the poverty of *expression* which occurs in parkinsonism, and from the dulling effects of other illnesses and of certain drugs. All these other conditions are potentially treatable.

Motivation

To a large extent motivation, the drive and energy to do things, depends on imagination, reasoning and emotions. But some patients are much more inactive and apathetic than expected. They seem to have a specific loss of motivation. Attempts to get them to 'get up and go' are frustrated and lesser goals have to be set. This can be one of the most disappointing aspects of dementia for optimistic energetic helpers. It may explain some cases of self-neglect or 'Diogenes syndrome' (p. 62). It must be distinguished from depression where the patient's low spirits make her disinclined to be active. And sometimes antidepressants (in America even amphetamine-like drugs) have been used in an attempt to improve motivation, usually with little success. Family or staff have to fill the gaps in motivation by using their own energy, but it can be a soul-destroying task.

Personality

Personality (p. 61) is really a mixture of many of the functions mentioned in this chapter — learnt social skills, attitudes and other characteristic ways of thinking, learnt habits of behaviour, typical emotional reactions and habitual reactions to various stresses. It goes without saying therefore that we can witness a gradual decline in all aspects of personality in dementia. This 'death of the personality' is most distressing for relatives (p. 189). It is important that staff who have never met the sufferer before get to know what she was like before the illness began, and do not assume that the rather dulled, blank person they meet is her original self. Again it is important to distinguish *apparent* decline due to depression, social withdrawal, physical illness or drugs from the real decline of dementia. *Change* in personality, where dementia causes *new* personality traits to emerge, is dealt with in the next chapter.

EXPRESSIONS AND ACTION

Speech problems

We have already (p. 94) seen the difficulties which dementing people have in *receiving* speech whether it be spoken or written. Often the 'central' processes of understanding meaning are more affected than the simple perception of words and grammar. We find something similar when we look at the *expression* of speech.

Even if a person has understood a question such as 'What did you have for breakfast?' and has enough memory to know the answer, there is still a very complex process to go through in order to produce an answer which will be fully understood. Some sense of the meaning to be got across is necessary; the right sounds and syllables must be used to construct the correct words, which then need to be assembled grammatically; this must then be translated into muscular action and actual expression.

Speech in dementia

Dysarthria. Eventually most of these aspects of speech will decline in dementia. The severely demented patient is often mute, or gives out only scattered inarticulate, meaningless fragments of speech. But till near the end the physical mechanism, the *articulation* of speech is usually quite normal. In MID, a particular stroke may affect the controlling centres of articulation, causing what is called *dysarthria*. Other neurological conditions, such as parkinsonism, can lead to disorders of articulation. But the simply demented person articulates speech quite normally.

Language. The difficulties for dementing people lie more in *language* than in speech. Indeed, the individual sounds, the syllables and words that result and even some simple aspects of grammar are relatively normal in earlier stages. It is the more complex processes of getting *meaning* across that decline first.

The result is that patients tend to use a smaller vocabulary and simpler, shorter sentences, and that they may become quite muddled when trying to get across more complex messages. Many also show a particular difficulty in *naming* objects and in naming lists of, for example, pieces of furniture or colours. These problems, which are akin to the problems of coding memories into 'boxes' have considerable effect on the patient's *fluency*. She will be frustrated in her attempts to get her meaning across and may try roundabout ways of describing things, called *paraphasia*. Her family find her speech both less interesting and more frustrating. It is little wonder that communication between the patient and her family declines. Nor is it surprising that patients come to rely on stock phrases, old stories and *platitudes* in their attempts to get some meaning across.

All these difficulties in expression will be made worse if the patient also suffers from *perseveration* (p. 128) or from a difficulty in excluding irrelevancies (p. 148), so that the clarity of her message gets lost because of repetitive or meaningless intrusions.

Dysphasias. Neurologists have defined specific dysphasias or difficulties with speech, both receptive and expressive, which are due to damage to quite specific areas of the brain. Occasionally an MID patient will show one of these specific dysphasias. However the speech problems of most dementing people are far too general to be defined so clearly. In one patient there will be some receptive dysphasia, much difficulty in comprehension and the formulation of meaning, some more specific expressive dysphasia, some loss of control, all mixed together. It is no wonder that speech therapists have tended to be pessimistic about helping dementing people, that the patients themselves tend to communicate less and less, and that relatives and friends are tempted to give up communicating with them. Only if one type of disorder predominates will specific help be possible.

Dysgraphia. A further problem which can arise is difficulty with writing, called *dysgraphia*, which can, for example, interfere with the patient's ability to remind herself of things by notes. It can be just as frustrating a problem as dysphasia.

Assessment

Speech and language problems are best assessed simply by listening to the patient speaking, either spontaneously or in answer to questions. Can she produce the right words, with the right grammar, does she get her meaning across, does she articulate properly? Or we may ask her to repeat some words back, to recite something she knows well, or to read. These tests show up expressive dysphasia. It is again important to judge how practically important her speech difficulties are. Do they mean that she cannot state her needs or are they merely frustrating?

Management

If someone has expressive problems but few receptive problems she will likely be frustrated by her inability to say clearly what she wants. We can lessen the frustration by guessing what she wishes to say. Relatives of dysphasic patients get very good at this guesswork, knowing that, for example, when she says something about going for a walk she wants the toilet. The relief for the patient in knowing that she is understood is enormous. Alternatively we can ask questions to find what she is trying to say. The forced choice technique is useful. 'Do you want the toilet or are you hungry?' In this way she gets across her meaning simply by a 'Yes' or 'No', or by a nod. A further method uses printed or written words. If she can point out the word that she needs she does not need to be able to say it properly.

On a more general level we should keep our sentences and questions to the patient simple. If we invite a complex answer it is unlikely to come clearly. Remember that poor short-term memory does not allow lots of material to be in her mind at once. And there is little value in letting the patient ramble on in an attempt to make sense, when she is losing sight of the subject and getting frustrated. It can be more helpful to inter-rupt and bring her back to the subject.

If there are more severe speech problems it may be useful to try to find other methods of communication. Touch and guidance by hand, pictures and photographs, and 'charades' which she can copy can all be helpful.

Unfortunately, as we have seen, many of the speech diffi-culties of dementing people are not of one sort or another, but are mixed. If she has difficulties in reception of speech, then our attempts to help her get over an expressive problem will be limited because she will not understand fully what we are saying. In MID there may be quite specific, single, speech difficulties and in such a case a speech therapist should be asked to give advice.

It is only when we see the effects of dysphasia that we see how important speech is in every aspect of everyday life. We should remember that not only does communication with others depend on speech but most of our internal thoughts are spoken. So that speech difficulties interfere fundamentally with the patient's ability to understand her situation, to solve problems and to think logically.

Co-ordinating action

The primary motor cortex (Fig. 1.2) is not affected in early ATD though in MID a stroke may affect this area or its connections. However, the motor cortex only controls the individual movements of muscles. The everyday actions that we carry out require interconnections with other regions of the brain, for they are complicated, involving different groups of muscles working together and depending on sensory input and learned habit. Actions such as dressing, going to the toilet, feeding, cooking all require very complex co-ordination. Impairment of this co-ordination is called *dyspraxia* and it is mainly due to damage in the parietal lobe. It usually goes along with agnosias and spatial disorientation as a common feature of ATD and it is often found in MID.

Dyspraxia may result in the patient *dressing* in the wrong order, putting her bottom clothes over her head, getting right and left mixed up, or being unable to manipulate buttons. She may have no problem of muscular weakness, stiffness or tremor but still be unable to carry out the essential actions of dressing. Similarly, dyspraxia can affect other activities, and we can quickly see how it leads to a need for outside help and to risks in the home. For the patient who is still at work, trying to carry out complex tasks becomes impossible.

Dyspraxia can be assessed by getting the patient to try to arrange play blocks in a particular pattern — showing what is called *constructional dyspraxia*. More practically, she can be asked to carry out various tasks of daily living. We need to be on the look-out for any other specific deficit like an agnosia, or right-left disorientation which is adding to the problem. For our aim is to fill in the specific gaps in the patient's ability as best we can. This means assessing not only what she cannot do, but what she can do. It may be, for example, that simply leaving out her clothes in order solves the problem of a dressing dyspraxia; it may be that we have to get each item the right way round for her to be able to put it on; or it may be that she only needs help with buttons. Simpler garments with Velcro fastening get round the problem at later stages, but in early stages the patient may feel better if she has been able to get 'proper' clothes on with only a little outside help. Almost all patients eventually need to be dressed and undressed completely. Similar remarks apply to the other actions which may be impaired by dyspraxia.

Mobility

Alzheimer-type dementia

Much of the need foir physical help with dressing, washing etc in ATD comes from the decline in learnt habits and from dyspraxia. The great majority of ATD sufferers remain otherwise remarkably physically fit till late stages of the illness. Major paralyses like strokes are not usually found, as they are in MID. However, as the disease progresses, patchy damage usually occurs in various parts of the *motor* system of the brain, those complicated pathways involved in the voluntary and involuntary control of muscles all over the body. The result may be some weakness of various muscles, some increase in muscle tone leading to reduced mobility and stiffness, or tremor and other abnormal movements. Eventually almost all patients show some of these changes. Because they are patchy and rather vague, it is difficult to decide on methods of treatment. The danger is that the patient's ability to walk independently can be lost. She is in danger of falling, loses her confidence and causes alarm in her carers. The result is that she may become chair- or bed-bound. These problems of mobility can also affect her use of her hands, eating and swallowing and all muscular movements.

Assessment. Other causes should always be considered before concluding that dementia is the cause of poor mobility, or other disorders of movement. Parkinsonism, stroke and the side-effects of drugs are all common causes. In particular, the phenothiazine drugs such as thioridazine can cause parkinsonian symptoms of muscular rigidity, tremor and poverty of movement. A shuffling gait with a tendency to take progressively smaller steps, difficulty in initiating movements, a blank, mask-like face, a regular tremor of the hands of 'pill-rolling' type, and excessive salivation should suggest parkinsonism due to Parkinson's disease or to these drugs. Other drugs cause mobility problems because of their sedative effects, because they lower blood pressure or because they cause tremor.

Management. In dealing with mobility problems, preventative action is best. Because of the tendency to withdraw socially the dementing patient may be inclined to sit in a corner 'not bothering anybody'. But this stores up physical problems for the future. Regular exercise can delay the decline in mobility. Relatives should be encouraged to take the patient out for a walk every day, for, besides its benefit as 'physiotherapy', this is stimulating for her and may reduce restlessness at other times. In group situations such as day care, residential home or hospital, the daily exercise group is important. It can be led by a physiotherapist, remedial gymnast, or any member of staff.

If there is a more specific problem such as localized weakness, rigidity or a tendency to fall, then referral to a physiotherapist is advisable, before the patient becomes too immobile. There are, of course, problems for dementing patients in physiotherapy. They may not understand the exercises they are asked to do, they may be dyspraxic or agnosic and use aids in the wrong way, they will be unlikely to be able to practice on their own. However, once a patient is chairfast, the situation can become irreversible. Muscles develop contractures through misuse and she will be unable to use her limbs properly ever again. There is also a danger of pressure sores. Passive exercises to prevent contractures and encourage freedom of movement are essential. However, not many patients will have access to enough physiotherapy time to carry out these treatments effectively. The physiotherapist should be prepared to instruct and advise nurses, care staff, and families in the principles of active physical rehabilitation and passive exercising. If immobility or contractures do develop, specialist physiotherapy should always be sought.

Walking aids — the stick, tripod and walking frame — are important aids, but like all gap-fillers should only be used if, after assessment, it is clear that the patient cannot cope at a higher degree of independence.

Falls. These can cause a great deal of anxiety to families and staff. They can of course be dangerous, and a significant number of dementing people suffer fractures of the femur and other bones. They are much more likely to do so if they are on sedative or other similar drugs, and mobility problems coupled with the patients' frequent carelessness contribute. The persistent wanderer is at risk if she has some degree of muscle weakness or other mobility problems. She is also at risk if she tires herself out. At the beginning of the day she may appear entirely fit, but by late afternoon she is 'falling on her feet'. The temptation is to confine her to a chair for her safety, for no-one likes to feel responsible if there is a risk and it has been ignored. But once confining to chair becomes a habit, the patient's mobility declines more rapidly. It is far better if staff or family can spare the time to walk her under supervision. A ward or home which does not have the staff to do this has too few staff (or the wrong sort of resident!). A family who cannot do this needs outside help.

Multi-infarct dementia

In addition to the problems just mentioned, which are likely to affect all dementia sufferers, MID patients may have more specific mobility problems. The strokes that they suffer can cause varying degrees of paralysis in one or other part of the body, ranging from minor weakness of one or two muscles, to hemiplegia — paralysis of one side of the body. The vast majority of strokes in MID, however, will not have any of these neurological manifestations, and will simply add to the general decline. Specific medical, nursing and physiotherapy attention will be required for any significant paralysis.

MID sufferers may also be more prone to other physical problems including 'funny tums', 'drop attacks', faints, dizziness, all of which lead to falls. Such episodes should not, however, be assumed to be simply part of the dementia, but deserve medical investigation.

Weight loss

Many patients lose considerable amounts of weight as their dementia progresses. This always demands medical investigation, but in most cases no medical cause is found. Uncoordinated swallowing may contribute, since it makes patients reluctant to eat for fear of choking. Forgetting to eat may also contribute, as may dyspraxia with eating utensils. But in many patients there is no such cause; they eat well but lose weight. There is a controlling mechanism for bodyweight in the centre of the brain which must be damaged by the dementia.

Indeed this may be part of that general, but vague, physical decline which leads eventually to the death of the sufferer.

CONCLUSION

Most dementing patients suffer most of the above losses to a greater or lesser degree. In MID the losses are often *patchy*, so that some of the more general functions, personality, emotional reactions or social skills are maintained till quite late in the dementia. In ATD, as well as the general losses there is concentration of damage in some temporal, frontal and parietal areas. But most patients eventually have most losses — dementia is truly a devastating condition.

The stages in the management of deficits and impairments in dementia can now be summarized:

1. Assess the loss
2. Assess what is left
3. Compare with past abilities
4. Assess the practical importance of the loss
5. Exclude causes other than dementia
6. Attempt retraining
7. Help the patient use her remaining abilities
8. Provide external help to fill the gaps
9. Do not take over completely until necessary.

This last point requires special emphasis. No loss can be considered complete until the last stage of the dementia. The patient is lo*sing* her abilities. Our chief aim should be to ensure that she uses what she still has as much as is reasonably possible, no more and no less.

5

Loss of control

So far we have considered dementia as a decline. And that
of course is basically what it is. But how can we explain the
fact that dementing people sometimes behave in ways they
never did before, and sometimes even seem like a different
personality? This is one of the most distressing facets of
dementia for relatives, especially if they have been in a close
relationship for many years. It is difficult enough to cope with
a relative who is chronically ill with an incurable disease, and
more difficult when this illness involves a decline in their
whole being as a person to a state of dependence on others.
But it is extremely difficult if at the same time the family has
to get used to totally new behaviour, or a new type of
relationship with a person they hardly recognize. A mild
mannered man, for example, may become irritable and
aggressive, a quiet lady become noisy and demanding. Why
do these changes occur? Many of these *new* experiences of
dementia can be explained as variants of a general disorder
of the function of the brain — *disinhibition* or *loss of control*.

Inhibition in the brain

The messages which pass from one nerve cell to another by
chemical transmitter (Fig. 1.3) are of two types — messages

123

which increase the likelihood of the second cell reaching the point where it fires electrically to send a message to yet another cell, and messages which reduce that likelihood. In other words, messages are either *excitatory* or *inhibitory*. All the workings of the central nervous system depend on the complicated interplay between millions of these two types of message passing between millions of cells.

On a larger scale we can define certain areas of the brain which seem to have a generally inhibitory effect on other areas. Much of the activity of the frontal lobes (Fig. 1.2) is of this type. Inhibition can affect the amount of information coming into the brain (sensory input), particularly how much of this information we are consciously aware of. It can also affect the output from the brain, for example, expression in speech and in emotion, as well as the behaviour of the person. Inhibition is likely also to be involved in controlling the interconnections of the brain and the processing of information, for example in thinking, judging and planning. And there are more physical, neurological aspects of inhibition. Because the brain is damaged so widely in dementia, it is not surprising that there is a loss of inhibitory control, as well as loss of the positive functions described in Chapter 4. The result is that more is experienced than would normally be experienced; things said or done that would normally not be said or done.

DISINHIBITION OF INPUT TO THE BRAIN

Attention

Only a tiny fraction of the information from our senses can be allowed to reach consciousness. If we perceived every bit of what was in our field of vision as equally important, if we consciously heard every sound around us all the time (people who wear hearing aids complain of something like this experience), if all the sensations in our body claimed our attention, we would be bombarded with a jumble of information which we could not disentangle. We have to filter out extraneous and unwanted information, and focus on what is immediately relevant.

This filtering process is a form of inhibition and is called attention. It is a function of those parts of the brain which are involved in consciousness, including the reticular activating system (p. 49) and the frontal lobes; it is closely linked to consciousness. We wake when someone calls our name, we become alert and attend to the voice. When we are less conscious it is more difficult to attend, whether the lowered consciousness is due to sleep, coma or the clouding of acute confusion (p. 49). The level of consciousness and its daily changes are not actually altered in dementia; patients are fully awake by day and sleep normally at night . But the ability to attend is often impaired. The dementing patient is thus easily *distracted* by irrelevant things in her surroundings — the filter is not working. Dementing people may also be able to hold fewer *bits* of information in attention at one time. This can easily be tested by 'digit span', the ability to attend to and repeat back a series of 3, 4, 5 or 6 numbers (many psychologists call this ability *short-term memory*).

'Stuck' attention. Once attention is gained, a dementing person may 'get stuck' on that object. It can be puzzling to see someone absolutely engrossed in some sound or sight which has little relevance at the moment.

In severe dementia the patient has little ability to focus attention at all. It may be impossible to get her to attend to a voice out of the jumble of sounds in a ward, as she may be visually distracted by all sorts of things around her, and by nothing in particular, or she may spend hours engrossed in 'stuck' attention.

Management

In practical terms, we must make more than usual effort to gain the attention of a dementing patient, we should simplify information, giving only one or two simple items rather than complicated material, we should make whatever we want the patient to attend to stand out clearly from its background, and we should lessen distractions as much as possible.

Hallucinations

Visual hallucinations, and to a lesser extent other types of hallucination, are characteristic of acute confusion (p. 50). Whenever visual hallucinations occur, particularly if they begin quite suddenly, this should be our first guess in diagnosis. However, hallucinations can occur in dementia.

The usual story is of a lady who is alone at home. She mentions visitors, but describes them as rather strange. They do not speak, they seem to appear from nowhere and disappear into thin air, or through the wall. She does not feel paranoid as they do not appear threatening. But she is bewildered and amazed, especially if she has made tea for them. She may realize that the experience is ridiculous and have partial insight, but the very real appearance of these visitors is likely eventually to convince her that she is not imagining them. This sort of experience usually occurs in early dementia, and often the patients involved also have eye problems such as cataract or glaucoma. It is possible that loneliness and the wish for companionship at a time of failing faculties may encourage imagination. However, it is likely that much of this phenomenon is due to a failure in the filtering out of irrelevant visual information by the brain. A similar sort of experience occurs when we walk along a very dark lane and shapes on the edge of our visual field seem like figures, or seem to move, and when we imagine we hear sounds in a silent house at night.

In more severe dementia, when there is a more severe breakdown of the attention process, when reality and imagination are less clearly differentiated, disorganised hallucinations occur. Patients may be observed talking to long dead relatives or to people who never existed. When asked, they can only vaguely describe whether they are seeing or hearing these people, or neither.

Detection. The detection of hallucinations is quite difficult, particularly in these later stages. Only if the patient can actually tell us of her experiences can we be sure. Often the only evidence is that she *seems* to be seeing things that are not real. It is easy to misunderstand hallucinations and describe what is happening as 'disorientation' or 'memory impairment' because the patient is preoccupied with her experiences, does not see them as abnormal, but acts oddly and appears out of touch with reality. The result is that she may appear to be more impaired than she actually is. So it is doubly important to check orientation, memory etc. in any patient with hallucinations.

Management. Firstly, the other signs and causes of acute confusion should be ruled out. Secondly, we should ensure that the patient's eyesight and hearing are checked and aided as much as possible. Thirdly, we should make the real environment stimulating, though simple, engaging her attention in ways that she can understand, with as few distractions as possible. Hallucinations are often worse at night when it is more difficult to make sense of what we see or hear. A night light is therefore advisable.

These measures may reduce the likelihood of hallucinations, but, once the hallucinations are established and firmly believed in, are unlikely to take them away completely. Drug treatment may therefore be necessary but only after the other measures have been tried. One of the antipsychotic drugs such as thioridazine, trifluoperazine or pimozide may help. But unfortunately drugs are not likely to be completely effective. It is unlikely that a large dose will do anything more than a small dose and may merely oversedate the patient.

Principles of management

For the dementing with disorders of attention or hallucinations we can begin to see some general principles which will apply to other disinhibitory phenomena:

— Look for *other causes.*
— Look at the *circumstances* in which the abnormalities occur. Can these be changed to lessen the problem?
— Can we *encourage more normal experience* and behaviour?
— *Drug treatment* is a last resort and should be used in smallish doses.

DISINHIBITION OF OUTPUT

Disinhibition in speech

We have considered in Chapter 4 the declines that occur in the various aspects of speech in dementia. The problem of focusing attention will apply to the spoken and the written word and therefore exacerbate problems of *comprehension*. But disinhibition may explain three other abnormalities that occur in the *expression* of speech, namely perseveration, 'stuck' speech and disinhibited content of speech.

Perseveration

This can be described as a difficulty in shifting from one subject to another. We have already seen something similar in relation to attention. Normally, when we answer a question, when we call someone's name, when we express something, we realize that we have said what is necessary and can prevent ourselves saying it again. We then move on to the next subject. This is, in fact, another controlling or inhibitory mechanism in the brain. I am not talking so much about that conscious social control, which prevents us from 'going on' about something when we see that others have got our message or are bored. This is to do with our personality, and our social awareness (p. 142). Perseveration is a much more basic problem which can make a person *unable* to shift from subject to subject. The controlling mechanism which is damaged in perseveration seems largely to be a function of the frontal lobes and we will see that the same applies to other inhibitory mechanisms affecting the output of the brain and the internal processing of information.

Perseveration in diagnosis. At the early stages of dementia, perseveration can be a very important diagnostic sign. It is most easily detected when we ask a series of questions of the patient — the time, the day, the date, the year, the patient's age. She may answer a question with the previous answer, even to the extent of getting stuck on the first answer and giving it for every question. Or parts of an answer may carry over to later answers, so that if the time is '11', the year becomes '1911'. The patient may or may not be aware of making these mistakes. People who do not suffer from any form of brain damage very seldom show evidence of perseveration. So it is a useful sign of organic brain disease, even when orientation, memory, and other brain functions are not greatly impaired.

Management. We should be aware of perseveration in

talking with dementing patients. We may have to move from subject to subject very slowly, or give a lot of extra clues to ensure that the patient has moved her whole attention onto the new subject. ('How old are you? We're talking about your age and how many years old you are. Do you understand?')

'Stuck speech'

At later stages, and occasionally early in dementia, more extreme forms of perseveration can occur. A word, a phrase or a story may get repeated over and over again as if a record was stuck — the 'gramophone sign'. If this happens in early dementia the patient may be aware of what they are doing but seem powerless to stop it. Later on they are less likely to be aware. The classical examples are patients in a ward who shout for a relative continually or cry 'Nurse, nurse, nurse' despite having no obvious physical or psychological distress. They continue this even when the relative or nurse is present and they cannot explain why they wanted them.

Management

Following the four principles mentioned above, we can work out how to attempt to treat this repetitiveness.

Other causes may be contributing. Real physical distress or unhappiness of any kind will naturally make the patient more likely to call for help, to the person who seems most likely to respond. If she forgets that the person has responded then she is likely to repeat the call for help. A thorough search for causes of distress or discomfort is therefore most important, before we start treating disturbed behaviour as due to loss of control.

Circumstances and environment. Even if a patient is repeating words or phrases during large parts of the day, it is unlikely that she is doing it all the time, or at the same intensity all the time. This variation in behaviour gives an opportunity to modify it by altering the circumstances.

The first step is to define the problem carefully and agree the definition among all concerned. If this is not done, people are recording and discussing slightly different problems. What type of speech is to be considered as repetitive?

Is it particular words? How many times does it have to be repeated to be considered repetitive? Is only shouted speech to be considered?

These and other clarifying questions prepare for the second step which is to record *when* it happens. This is best done using a *behavioural chart* (Table 5.1). The first type involves observing when her behaviour is most obvious and recording the circumstances. This is most appropriate for recording things which a patient does relatively seldom, such as being incontinent, so it is less useful in a case of repetitiveness than the second type. This involves time sampling. No-one is going to be able to record every instance of very repetitive behaviour. So either a record can be kept of what the patient is doing, say, every hour on the hour; or she can be observed more closely for, say, quarter hour periods at various times of the day. The circumstances to be recorded include, 'What time of day is it?', 'What else is the patient doing?', 'Is she engaged in activity or not?', 'Where are other people in relation to her?', 'What relatives or staff are around?', 'How do other people *react* to her behaviour?'

From the chart, a pattern will probably emerge. Perhaps it is seen that she behaves in the undesirable way with staff but not with relatives. The behavioural chart can then be modified to look more closely at the type of interactions that occur and particularly at how the two groups of people react to her shouting. Then by altering the circumstances, the behaviour may be modified and lessened. And this is true even though the damage to the control systems in the brain is an organic change which cannot be reversed.

Behaviour modification is most effective if we can identify something which has been *rewarding* or *encouraging* the patient's behaviour. If when she shouts she always get attention, that attention may actively encourage her to shout more. Attention may consist of a kind word, physical contact, something that is thought to be pleasing such as a sweet, or something to read to divert her attention from the shouting. Even a 'telling off' is a form of attention. Attention can come from family, staff and other residents and is usually given with very good motives. So withdrawing these rewards can sometimes seem cruel. However it is often effective. If a lady is calling for help it is easy to feel obliged to go, even if we are almost

Table 5.1

Type 1 (This patient has only occasional episodes)			
Time of noisy episode	Circumstances	Reactions of Staff	Outcome
9.15 a.m.	After breakfast, alone by bedside	Asked to join others in day room	A bit quieter
1.05 p.m.	After lunch, sitting by bedside	Ignored	Later seen joining others
4.00 p.m.	Relatives have just left	Told that relatives would return	Remained noisy for 1 hour then stopped

This patient was only disturbed when 'left alone'.

Type 2 (This patient has very frequent episodes)			
Time sampled	Number of noisy episodes	Where was patient?	Who was around?
9 - 9.15 a.m.	1	Bedroom	Alone, nurse nearby with another patient
11 - 11.15 a.m.	3	Day room	In exercise group
1 - 1.15 p.m.	2	Dining room	With 5 patients at table
3 - 3.15 p.m.	0	Day room	With relatives

This patient was more disturbed when with other patients.

certain that she is crying 'wolf'. But it may be important to stop going in order to lessen very distressing behaviour.

Consistency is important in carrying out such a 'behaviour modification' programme. If some relatives or staff are prepared to carry through a programme which means lessening their response to calls for help while others are not, the programme is unlikely to be very successful. Continuing the charts during the 'treatment' is an important check on consistency. But more important is to get everybody's agreement beforehand that they are prepared to be consistent in their approach. Unfortunately, such behaviour modification programmes are often sabotaged by relatives, or by well meaning domestic staff, or, most often of all, by other residents, dementing or not, who cannot stop themselves reacting in a normal 'helpful' way when a patient seems to be distressed. A lot of explanation and support is needed throughout a behaviour modification programme if it is to succeed. Much depends on the persistence and enthusiasm of the person in charge of the programme.

Furthermore, taken to extremes, such programmes *can* be cruel, if they involve completely ignoring patients or 'time out' and other techniques that are near to punishment. The dementing patient will be unable to understand what is going on and may be put under considerable unwarranted stress. The need to involve all relatives and staff and the need to keep a programme under review should prevent such excesses and make sensible behaviour modification more effective.

Occasionally much of this effort is unneeded. The extra general attention to the patient and the fact that staff have to record their own responses are sufficient in themselves to bring an improvement in the problem. The difficulty then becomes one of maintaining improvement.

Encouraging normal behaviour. The behavioural chart will show times when the patient is quiet, perhaps during mealtimes, perhaps when visitors come, perhaps in the morning, perhaps when others in a day room are quiet. The other side of reducing attention when she is noisy is to increase attention when she is not, so encouraging her to be quiet for longer periods. Once again, an examination of the behaviour chart may show which factors encourage quietness. These can then be increased. Most commonly, attention and physical contact given at quiet times or engagement in activities will be helpful. Increasing attention at these other times will help family or staff feel less unhappy about reducing attention at the noisy times.

The sort of attention or 'reward' that is given, should be chosen for the individual patient. It should be rewarding specifically for her. Not everybody likes physical contact, or the chance to go out and about, or sweets, and some people are rewarded by quite 'odd' things, like being alone, being allowed to go to bed, or listening to music or television programmes which others do not like. The timing of reward and attention is also important. Especially for dementing people, rewards cannot be delayed, for the patient will forget and the link between what they are doing and the encouragement gets lost. There is no point in promising a reward later; it has to be given at the time.

The clinical psychologist is the expert in behavioural techniques, and will help in devising charts, planning treatment programmes, continuing supervision, and discussing any difficulties which arise.

Drug treatment. This is the last resort. As I have already said, it is unlikely that a big dose will bring more effect than a small dose, and oversedation is the likely consequence of overdosing. The choice of drug has to be by trial and error. The drug which works is the best one. It may be a phenothiazine such as thioridazine or promazine, it may be haloperidol or droperidol, it may be a benzodiazepine drug such as oxazepam. The benzodiazepine drugs can occasionally actually cause disinhibition so they must be used with caution. And phenothiazines can cause restlessness (called akathisia) which can be mistaken for a worsening of the behaviour problem.

All this being said, it is also important to remember that the abnormalities in behaviour that I am describing are due to organic damage, if other causes have been ruled out, and so the chances of total success are by no means great. Nevertheless an improvement in repetitive shouting which makes a dementing lady more tolerable to live with and avoids having to send her to long-stay hospital care is worth considerable effort. And working out a treatment programme, rather than assuming that nothing can be done, transforms our attitude to the dementing patient.

Disinhibited content of speech

Since this is akin to other problems of social behaviour we will discuss it under that heading (p. 140).

Emotional disinhibition

The ability to control emotions varies from person to person and is an important aspect of personality. Some people are impulsive, some irritable, some easily moved to tears, some placid, some over-controlled in their emotions. But we are all capable of a wide range of emotional reactions. Even the coolest person is aware that they could, if they 'let go', be much more openly emotional, and even the most emotional person does not express everything that they feel. The mechanism of emotional control is again a function mainly of the frontal lobes and their connections, and so is likely to be impaired in all forms of dementia, but particularly if there is a lot of damage in the frontal area.

Two main types of problems can occur: emotional lability and 'stuck' emotions.

Emotional lability

Labile means 'prone to change easily'. Emotional lability is changeability of one or more than one emotion. What happens is that something causes an emotional response which would usually be fairly minor, for example, the mention of the patient's long dead father. Instead of her normal, slight sadness on thinking of him, an emotion which is under control, she loses control and bursts into floods of tears. Likewise a tiny argument with her husband can lead the patient to an outburst of anger, out of all proportion to the cause, and even end in physical aggression. And other emotions — fear or laughter for example — can be involved. The swing of emotion usually starts very suddenly, within a few seconds, and there is just as sudden a recovery. What is more, the patient may have complete insight. In other words, she realizes that her reaction has been excessive, cannot explain why it has happened, and is full of embarrassment at her behaviour.

An extreme form of emotional lability has been called the *'catastrophic reaction'*. Here the patient has been subjected to a series of questions in rapid succession or has been posed a complicated problem or otherwise 'overloaded' mentally. Having lost the skill to ask for more time or give herself space to think she begins to be upset. Lability of emotion then brings a very sudden burst of severe emotion, whether tears, fear or anger, which brings the interview to an end.

Management of lability

Using our principles of management of disinhibition we can often help emotional lability to some extent.

Other causes. We must first ensure that the emotions expressed are not due to some other cause; that they are not real emotional reactions to a difficult situation (Ch. 6) or the outcome of disturbed relationships with family or staff (Ch. 7), and that the lability is not due to acute confusion or to the effects of drugs such as benzodiazepines or anti-parkinsonian drugs.

Circumstances. Using a behavioural chart the pattern and circumstances of the lability can be recorded after clearly defining the problem. The type of chart on which each episode of disturbed behaviour is recorded (Table 5.1) is more often useful here, since episodes of lability are often quite widely scattered over time. The factors which are causing the lability to occur may well include circumstances which 'raise the emotional temperature'. Even quite severely demented patients can be sensitive to the emotional atmosphere long after their ability to express feelings in words is lost. People who meet a dementing patient will vary greatly in the degree of calmness or emotional expression with which they react to her. Those who are anxious about the patient, upset by her, frustrated by her, or confrontative will induce an emotional reaction which, in the absence of proper control, can lead to a labile response. Other exacerbating factors may include situations which bewilder or frustrate the patient — confusing surroundings, too many questions, too much choice, or situations which will show up her disabilities.

Having identified the exacerbating factors we can look into ways of modifying them. We may need to teach each other how to be calm with the patient, or we may need to simplify her surroundings and activities, to avoid frustrations where possible.

A most distressing vicious circle can develop if a relative or staff member assumes that the patient's emotional response is intentional. If, for example, a dementing wife becomes angry in a disinhibited way with her husband he may feel that she is getting at him and react just as strongly back. Or a relative may try to shout down the patient who is getting emotionally upset, instead of lowering the emotional temperature. These reactions disturb the patient even more and the whole situation can get out of hand, even ending in violence. It does not take a chart to see what is happening. But if the relative's excessive reaction to the patient has been a lifelong habit it will be very difficult to get him to change. Often the only thing which helps is for the relative to leave the room for a while until both settle down.

This sort of over-reaction by relatives shows up very clearly if the patient attends day care or goes into respite care. A problem of emotional lability at home turns out to be no problem in the other setting. Partly this is because people are on their best behaviour' when they go among strangers. But partly it is because of a different emotional 'level'. Unfortunately the ordinary, warm emotional bond between husband and wife can be enough to increase the likelihood of lability, without anything being wrong in their relationship. This is one of the reasons why caring husbands or wives need a regular break. But it is also worthwhile spending effort in trying to teach a relative how to distance themselves emotionally from the patient — learning how to 'cool it'.

Normal behaviour. The 'normal' times when the patient is not labile give clues as to what helps her feel at ease. This is likely to be a calm, non-frustrating, non-bewildering environment. There is little more that can be done to encourage these settled times. The treatment of lability consists mainly of reducing the labile episodes.

Drugs. Once again the choice of drugs is wide and trial and error must be used. Sometimes an anti-depressant drug may be helpful if the patient is generally in low mood as well as suffering episodes of labile tearfulness or other distress. But more often a small dose of a phenothiazine or similar drug helps best.

'Stuck' emotions

Here the ups and downs of emotion are lost and the patient seems unable to move away from a particular emotion. Thus she may be constantly anxious for no apparent reason, or persistently irritable, or spend long parts of the day in tears. The curious dissociation between emotional expression and actual subjective feeling which occurs in lability may also apply here. So, in contrast to someone suffering from depression, the tearful lady may say that she does not know what is upsetting her, or even that she feels perfectly happy. In other patients a search for meaning makes them identify some cause for their emotion. Needless to say this cause may be quite imaginary. If the emotion is sadness, she may complain that a parent has gone away, or that she is going to die. If it is anger, she may make a paranoid interpretation, that someone is getting at her. If it is anxiety, she invents a danger of fire, harm to relatives etc.

More common than these distressing emotions, though, is 'stuck' happiness, a state of vacuous euphoria which is the permanent emotion of many dementia sufferers. To some extent this is due to the gradual loss of all other emotions (p. 112), but at the end of this decline patients often seem positively happy, and certainly happier than they might be expected to be, suffering such a dreadful illness as dementia. There must be an element of disinhibition as well.

Management

Management of these disorders of mood is quite difficult. Euphoria is usually seen as a blessing rather than a disorder, and few would wish to 'cure' it by presenting the awful truth of their condition to the happy sufferers. And it is difficult to estimate how subjectively distressed patients with other 'stuck' emotions are. Do they actually *feel* the emotions or not? Even if they do not feel distressed, or forget that they have been like this for months, it must be a bewildering condition to be in, and, of course, it is extremely distressing for relatives and others to see the patient apparently in severe and constant distress.

The behavioural approach is worth trying, but often does not identify clear causes. Distracting the patient into other engaging activities can be very helpful but even in the new activities the emotions may return, upsetting other people around her. Often drug treatment must be used, trying to match the drug to the emotional state — an anti-anxiety drug for anxiety, an anti-depressant for depression, a phenothiazine or similar drug for anger, especially if associated with paranoid thinking. Once again the choice is made by trial and error, but bigger doses of drugs may be required than in lability. However, as before, success cannot be guaranteed and a few patients have to survive in this apparently distressed state for long periods.

The period of disturbance eventually comes to an end in most cases. This is because the decline of the dementia eventually affects the ability to feel or express any emotion at all. So the emotional disturbance dies away. Both lability and 'stuck' emotions are more often (though not always) problems of early and moderate dementia. Indeed this is a general rule of disinhibition in dementia, that *the problem is likely to be worse in earlier stages and to lessen as the dementia becomes more severe.*

Disinhibited behaviour

A lot of the experience and activity that we have been discussing in attention, speech and emotion has been learnt. And many of the controls or inhibitory mechanisms in the brain are also learnt. When we turn to social behaviour (how people interact with other people and how they behave in relation to the 'rules' of society), a great deal of learning over many years must be involved in order to develop a sense of what is 'right' in a particular situation and what is 'wrong'. By Ribot's law, we would expect loss of social controls to be quite an early problem in dementia. Indeed it can be the first sign.

The frontal lobes are the main site of control of behaviour, and functions such as conscience, social awareness, self-control, moral ideas and judgement seem to be largely carried on in this part of the brain and through its connections. Damage leads to a decline in this learnt control resulting in disinhibited behaviour. And, since much of our description of personality depends on how a person behaves socially, it is these changes which are usually meant when families talk of a dementia sufferer having a *'change of personality'*.

We use a wide range of controls and inhibitions in our behaviour from day to day. These will vary from person to person. We all know people who have more or less social graces, or have more or less concern for right or wrong than others. These are personality differences. In dementia we are interested in a *change* from the individual's normal, so it is most important to get an account of her previous personality from a relative, before suggesting that a particular individual is showing behaviour disorder. We must always beware of imposing *our* standards of behaviour on other people. Even more important, we must beware of an institution inventing a set of standards for its own convenience and treating anything different as abnormal. A person who has always been sloppy at the table, or used swear words, or been light fingered with others' property is unlikely to change into a perfect resident when she is dementing (unless the dementia takes away her drive to do these things, or unless she anyway had a more 'correct' public facade). Let us look at examples of various forms of disinhibited behaviour before examining ways of managing 'problem' behaviour.

Perseveration of action

The sort of difficulty of moving from one subject to another, mentioned above under speech, can occur also in relation to actions. The patient who tries to change from one action (say, pouring the tea) to another (say, adding sugar) finds herself unable to do so, and ends up pouring tea into the sugar bowl. She may or may not be aware of the problem.

Old habits

An interesting phenomenon which is due to disinhibition is

the reappearance of old habitual actions, usually an action which was used at work. Such actions have been learnt and repeated many, many times over years, but may have last been performed 20 years or more previously. Loss of inhibition allows their return. This usually causes no problem, but may be a great puzzle until an old workmate or a relative recalls its original meaning. Repetitive dusting actions may even be put to some present use!

Rituals

New repetitive actions may also emerge. The failure of control allows a repetitive habit to continue and become established. Such rituals as turning on and off taps (sometimes with disastrous consequences), folding pieces of paper or touching certain objects are quite common. They may have arisen out of early reactions of the patient to her dementia (Ch. 6), particularly from attempts to keep a crumbling world in order with reminders or routine, but they become fixed and meaningless.

Conversation

Unnecessary or meaningless words can get into speech by loss of the normal inhibitory mechanisms. However, the content of our speech is also controlled by our understanding of what is proper, what is acceptable content to the person we are talking to. Loss of this inhibition may lead a polite lady to start using swear words, or a careful lady to say just what she thinks about someone else. Sometimes the *amount* of speech is affected and someone who was very quiet speaks endlessly.

Table manners

A coarsening of table manners is often seen in dementia, ranging from being sloppy to eating everything in sight (even including the soap and the houseplants).

Dressing and undressing

Normally how we dress depends on the standards of those

of our own sex, age and social group. Some dementing
people, quite apart from their declining ability to dress properly (p. 118) or remember to change their clothes, seem to
choose to wear eccentric clothes. They seem to have lost the
concern for their own appearance which is part of our social
relationships. In other cases the problem is one of undressing
in public, the patient losing her usual concern about privacy
and propriety. She may go out half-dressed or undressed in
the street, or undress in front of other residents. Undressing
can be an extreme problem, the patient dressing and
undressing repeatedly for no apparent reason. The most likely
cause is physical or mental distress on top of some disinhibition. The patient may be too hot. She may be uncomfort-
able because of incontinence, a desire to urinate, or
constipation. She may feel unwell or be made restless by
drugs. She may be anxious, depressed, or frustrated. She
may, of course, be particularly frustrated by a dressing
dyspraxia. But occasionally there is no exacerbating cause.

Excreting

Children learn quite early in life that it is considered correct
to urinate or defaecate in a toilet. If this learned social control
is lost, then anywhere will do. We should, however, separate
this type of inappropriate excretion, firstly from ignorance of
where the toilet is and therefore having to go somewhere
else, which will be highly embarrassing to the patient;
secondly from urgency, a need to rush to the toilet, but
perhaps not get there in time, caused by bladder problems;
and thirdly from true incontinence where *physical* control of
urination or defaecation has been lost (though this is also a
form of disinhibition — see p. 149). Of course many
dementing patients lose their conscience about these other
causes of 'accidents' and do not feel embarrassed by them as
a normal person would.

Physical contact

Social taboos prevent people from picking their noses or
touching their own genitals in public. They limit the amount
that people touch each other both sexually and non-sexually.

Older people in general do accept ordinary touching much more readily than younger people, perhaps because some of the sexual meaning of touch has been lessened. But in dementia the taboos may be lost. The good side of this is that touch can be used to help dementing people, to reassure and support them, to calm or to help engage them in activity. The not so good side is that patients may look for sexual contact in a disinhibited way. The worst situation of all arises when the object of sexual desire is apparently a completely new one, for example a happily married man who begins to show a disinhibited sexual interest in children.

Respect for others' possessions

When this inhibition is lost (partly due to a loss of the ability to recognize what is one's own), the patient may lift other people's belongings without concern. Mildly dementing people at home may become shoplifters. In a residential home or hospital a hoard of other people's possessions may be found in one resident's locker.

Asking for attention

In the section on speech (p. 129) we discussed repeated calls for help that are meaningless and due simply to a 'stuck' word. A more general change can occur whereby the patient loses the patience to wait for help, and becomes insistent, demanding of attention, even histrionic in her demands. Linked with some disinhibition of emotion, this can change a polite, patient, uncomplaining lady into a rather unattractive, cantankerous 'old woman' who demands immediate attention for real or imaginary complaints and who loses her temper, or acts out physical or mental distress if her demands are not met.

Restlessness

There are a number of different causes of restlessness in dementia which must always be considered (Table 5.2). Disinhibition is only one, and often indeed more than one type of cause applies. The other types of cause are physical

Table 5.2 Restlessness

Cause	Management
Physical discomfort e.g. pain, constipation, heat	Find cause and treat it
Acute confusion	Find cause (Table 2.3) and treat
Drug side-effect (akathisia)	Reduce drug
Need of customary exercise	Exercise
Searching for familiar territory	Reality orientation (RO)
Distress	
anxiety	Reassurance, RO, drugs
depression	Supportive psychotherapy, drugs
frustration	Assess losses, fill gaps
Disinhibition	Behaviour management, drugs

discomfort, physical illness, acute confusion, drug side-effects and emotional distress (including searching for familiar territory, anxiety, depression and frustration). Only when all of these have been ruled out should disinhibition as a sole cause of restlessness be considered.

Our activity is usually set at a particular general level, though where this controlling function is located in the brain is not known. There are of course variations, some people feeling active and energetic in the mornings, others in the afternoon, some feeling less inclined to be active as it comes to night-time in preparation for sleep. I have mentioned before the decline in activity and apathy which affects the majority of dementia sufferers (p. 113). For a minority, however, the opposite occurs. They lose the normal control and have an increase in their energy and activity. As with ritual behaviour, some of this may arise from early distress but the disturbed behaviour gets 'stuck'. In its extreme forms this overactivity, like mania or akathisia (general restlessness of the muscles) due to phenothiazine and related drugs, can appear unstoppable. The patient is unable to concentrate on anything or to relax for any length of time and seems to need to be in constant motion. Sleep may be lost and sitting long enough to have a meal becomes a problem.

More common than this constant overactivity is the change

in the usual diurnal variation in activity mentioned on page 90. For reasons which are obscure, the patient is settled throughout the morning, but beginning in late afternoon there is a build-up of restlessness until sleep comes. Relatives frequently report the disruption that this can bring to family life. Or they complain that day care is provided at the most settled part of the day. And staff who only work in the morning and early afternoon wonder why evening and night staff are complaining.

Management of behavioural disinhibition

Most of the steps in management have already been covered in the four principles on page 127, though some additional principles apply particularly to social disinhibition.

Other causes. Acute confusion, and particularly certain drug reactions, should be ruled out before deciding that disturbed behaviour is due to disinhibition. Among drugs, we should consider antiparkinsonian drugs such as L-dopa and bromocriptine which can be potent causes of restlessness, sexual disinhibition and other behaviour disorders, as well as causing confusion. Depression (p. 57) can cause restlessness and agitation. Mania (p. 60) can lead to disinhibited behaviour of all sorts and needs to be differentiated very carefully from dementia.

Identify the problem. The first questions to be asked are 'Is this behaviour posing a real problem? Does it upset the patient or does it upset others? If it is other people who are upset, is that because they have an intolerant attitude which might be changed?' This sort of questioning should be going on as we attempt to define the exact nature of the problem in its simplest terms.

Attitudes to disinhibition. It is important to look further at our attitudes towards the behaviour that is released by social disinhibition. We all know of things that we would like to do if only we were less inhibited. But it is not fair to the demented to assume that the disinhibited things they do are 'naughty' things that they have wanted to do for years and are now released. People are *capable* of behaving in all sorts of ways that they have never even thought of. It may be tempting in retrospect to see a lady's disturbed behaviour as a protest at past over-control. But this is only our fantasy unless we have real evidence that she actually wanted to act in a more disinhibited way. We should be tolerant of disinhibited behaviour in dementia, for it is due to organic brain disease and the patient cannot help what she is doing, but we should not encourage it because it is colourful, or seems rebellious.

External controls. Disinhibited social behaviour can be seen as due to a loss of conscience. Can we fill this gap by an external conscience? For we behave 'properly' not only because of our internal conscience, but also because others show disapproval if we behave 'improperly'. In dementia the ability to understand and respond to external disapproval or advice is gradually being lost so it may have little effect, especially in later stages of the illness. But it is worth consideration.

What I am suggesting is simply that if the patient has lost the ability to say 'No, don't do it' to herself, then someone else should say it to her. There is a danger, however, that we may become too punishing. The decision to use external control should therefore be based on very careful assessment. Will she understand what is being said? Does this external control make her embarrassed, guilty or frightened, by making her realize what she is doing 'wrong'? Does it make her angry or resentful without affecting her behaviour much? Or does it have to be done so often or so strongly that it causes 'overload' and a catastrophic emotional reaction? Do other patients and visitors understand what is being done and do they approve? Most important of all, does the attempt at external control actually encourage the behaviour it is supposed to stop?

All this being said, there is a definite place for external control. It is used by relatives, but they often feel quite guilty about what seems like scolding their spouse or mother. It is used by staff in hospitals and homes to control eating habits, or undressing in public, inappropriate urination or sexual misbehaviour. It should never be done in bad temper. And it should not be used willy-nilly on all patients. It is better decided upon after full discussion among everybody who is working with the particular patient.

Circumstances. Charting the circumstances of the patient's abnormal behaviour and others' reactions to it can again be very useful in identifying factors which make it happen more often. For antisocial interactions, the most important factors are likely to concern *who* the patient behaves towards in a disinhibited way, and *what response* she gets from them. Further, the response which reinforces her behaviour may not be the obvious one. We might expect that anger or disgust would stop undesirable behaviour. Paradoxically, such reactions can actually encourage it, probably because they represent some sort of interaction and so fulfil a basic human need. This is particularly a problem when there is little interaction at all with the patient except an occasional 'Stop that!'. Thus attempts at external control of the behaviour may actually have to be discouraged. Often, though, it is more general attention which has been reinforcing. People only notice her when she is doing something odd or startling and automatically pay more attention during these times. Withdrawing attention, rather than changing from being nice to being nasty, will be most helpful. But, of course, there may be protests, both from the patient and from relatives, other patients or staff who see the withdrawal of attention as dereliction of duty, especially if the patient is being antisocial.

Normal behaviour. In some cases it is possible to retrain patients to a limited extent. Sloppy habits in eating or dressing are likely to be most easily helped this way. In general, encouragement, praise and reinforcement appropriate to the individual should be tried. It should be given immediately after the patient has properly performed what at other times she does in a disinhibited way. Again success is likely to be limited. But a combination of reducing reinforcement of abnormal behaviour and positive reinforcement of more normal behaviour, together with judicious use of external controls, can bring enough improvement to change an undesirable, unpopular patient into a more acceptable and likeable person who has a better quality of life.

Some of this change will have been brought about by changing circumstances. But some assumes an ability to learn, for behaviour therapy is largely based on theories of learning. The improvement achieved by any of these techniques must be limited by the declining ability of the patient to learn

(p. 109). Indeed, at later stages of dementia, learning ability is so slowed as to be effectively absent. Furthermore the patient's ability to make or receive any meaningful contact with the outside world is declining. So behaviour modification is likely to be less effective later on. On the other hand, behaviour and experience are often simpler at the later stages, so simple modifications of circumstances can occasionally bring surprisingly good results. The most obvious examples of this occur when a demented lady moves from one environment to another, or when she becomes physically ill. Behaviour which has been disinhibited and troublesome in one set of circumstances can disappear overnight. The lesson is that behaviour modification should always be given a chance.

Maintaining improvement. If behaviour has improved, there is always a tendency to relax and fall back into old ways of responding. Whoever is in charge of a behaviour programme should ensure that its principles are continued, and should remind family or staff from time to time of what has helped. If the behaviour returns, a repeat programme may be justified.

Drugs. The same principles apply as before. As a last resort small doses of phenothiazine drugs may help to control disinhibited behaviour. An apparent improvement that is merely caused by oversedation is undesirable. The oversedated patient is likely to be more confused, less physically able, and less able to co-operate — a combination which will add to rather than lessen the difficulties of her behaviour.

DISINHIBITION OF THINKING

I have earlier described the usual poverty of thinking of dementia sufferers (p. 111). But often we come across odd or quite bizarre ways of thinking among patients. Some of these are caused by attempts to make sense of what is happening (p. 181) in the absence of proper information from senses or memory. But the fact that the patient seems to accept these peculiar ideas as normal requires some further explanation.

Within our minds thoughts are judged by a standard of acceptability that we learn. We treat whatever is not accepted in a variety of ways — as dreaming, as imagination, as contradictory, as something that it is not polite to think. If this controlling mechanism is not present, then previously unacceptable thoughts become acceptable, and unacceptable thoughts are not dismissed.

Often a patient will hold ideas that *contradict* each other, or contradict reality. An example is the person who says that her parents are alive and yet also knows that she herself is 85. This 'double orientation' is partly due to memory loss, but there must be an absence of something inside her, saying 'That must be nonsense'. If such contradictory thoughts become fixed she can be said to suffer from a *delusion*, which cannot be shifted by reason. She is absolutely convinced that her parents are alive. This type of loss of judgement contributes to the paranoid delusions which some dementing people develop to explain their memory lapses (p. 181).

In most patients however the odd ideas do not become fixed, and they may be held for very brief times. Some *illusions*, in which the patient misinterprets what she sees or hears (see also p. 50) are due to faulty judgement, as well as showing poor perception.

Perseveration of thinking and '*stuck*' thoughts also occur. The extreme of this is *obsessional* thinking, in which the patient is forced, against her will, to think the same thought again and again. More often there is a simple difficulty in moving from one thought to another, so that clear thinking becomes very difficult.

Another aspect of this sort of controlling mechanism of thoughts is *planning*, which is used to build up complicated courses of action and to prevent us from rushing into things. We have already seen one example of lack of planning in relation to people who behave in a demanding way (p. 142), wanting immediate responses, rather than seeing that a more planned and organized request for help might be more effective.

Problems of planning and judgement affect the patient's ability to understand her current circumstances and make rational decisions (Ch. 8). There is little that can be done to recover the power of judgement once it is lost. Presenting facts in a simple way and reinforcing reality by repetition can help; but drug treatment may be needed if the patient is deluded and decision-making may have to be taken away from the patient if her thinking becomes out of touch with reality.

NEUROLOGICAL DISINHIBITION

The theory of how disinhibition can cause symptoms is largely due to Hughlings Jackson, an American neurologist of the last century. He saw the brain as divided into less advanced 'lower' parts and more advanced 'higher' centres. The latter had a largely controlling function over the former so that when higher centres were damaged, one result would be loss of this control and the emergence of more primitive functions. Looking at disinhibited social behaviour as an example, we can see that this theory fits quite well. We learn with our 'higher' frontal bits of the brain (parts that are much smaller in 'lower' animals) to control our social behaviour. Loss of frontal lobe function means that 'lower', less advanced types of functioning re-emerge.

Jackson's experience, however, was neurological. For example, damage to the frontal lobes can lead to the emergence of primitive reflexes such as the sucking reflex and the grasp reflex which usually are only present for a short time after birth and then disappear. They have been inhibited during all those intervening years, but the possibility of them occurring has remained, and is released by the loss of inhibition.

Incontinence

The commonest neurological disinhibition in dementia, however, is incontinence. From the base of the frontal lobes, an inhibitory mechanism passes down the spinal cord to the bladder, preventing it from opening. Normally this can only be overcome by the voluntary decision to urinate, and of course we are reminded of the need to do this by messages coming up from the bladder which indicate that it is full. If the inhibition from the brain is lost, then the bladder may empty without voluntary control. A somewhat similar, though less sophisticated, mechanism controls defaecation.

In dementia sufferers there are a number of ways in which inappropriate urination and defaecation occur, not all of which are true incontinence. The true loss of control incontinence of dementia should occur relatively late in the progress of the disorder and urinary incontinence should occur before faecal incontinence, according to Ribot's law (p. 7). So incontinence occurring earlier in dementia is more likely to be due to other causes. There is one exception. In normal pressure hydrocephalus (p. 29), loss of control incontinence occurs early in the course of the illness.

Urinary incontinence

The types of incontinence of urine met with in dementing patients are:

1. Incontinence due to a *urinary tract infection*. When incontinence starts, especially if it occurs suddenly and if there are symptoms of an infection — discomfort during urination, pain in the lower abdomen or loin, raised temperature — a midstream specimen of urine must be taken and checked for infection. Urinary infections are usually treatable, though recurrence is a problem, especially in women. If continence has been lost because of an infection it usually returns after treatment, but a little retraining may be necessary. It is not clear to what extent urinary infections *without* symptoms cause incontinence.

2. Incontinence of urine due to *constipation*. The mass of faeces in the rectum disrupts the mechanics of urination and can lead to incontinence of urine. This will improve after the constipation is relieved.

3. *Diuretic treatment* can lead to or exacerbate incontinence. In particular a diuretic drug given later in the day can give rise to night incontinence, and the night-time cup of tea can make things worse still. Diuretics should be given in the morning, in the mildest form and the lowest dose that are absolutely necessary. Unfortunately these are very widely used drugs and patients tend to continue taking them for years with little review.

4. *Self-neglect incontinence*. The patient who has withdrawn and become depressed or apathetic may not bother about her self-care and gradually become incontinent. Social

stimulation and improved morale can reverse this.

5. *Incontinence due to loss of 'conscience'.* The patient with frontal lobe type of damage loses social concern, and may urinate in inappropriate places. This is a form of disininhibited behaviour needing behavioural management (p. 141), and is not a neurological disinhibition.

6. *Inability to get to the toilet.* Memory impairment and disorientation leave the patient unable to find the toilet, and, especially if they suffer *urgency* or *frequency* of micturition, incontinence is the result. Poor mobility leads to the same problem. Anxiety and embarrassment result, and can make urgency worse and so by a vicious circle, increase the incontinence. Good signposting and a regular toileting programme to suit the particular patient can cure this problem. The poorly mobile patient, or the patient who suffers urgency will feel much more relaxed if they can sit within sight of a toilet. At night the provision of a commode or a bottle or bedpan can avoid considerable problems (though the patient has to remember that these aids are there!). It is important to learn just how the patient feels, complains or behaves when she needs to urinate, especially if she is unable to say directly and needs help to get to the toilet.

7. In women, symptoms of *stress incontinence* and the related problems of vaginal prolapse can range from the passage of small amounts of urine when the patient coughs to severe loss of control. Symptoms are likely to have been present long before the onset of the dementia, but may be exacerbated by one or other of the factors above. Gynaecological help is required to treat this.

8. In men, incontinence may be related to *prostate* enlargement. The most common problem is frequency of micturition by day and night, the patient passing small quantities of urine with difficulty, but very often. If there is a problem of finding the toilet, this can easily lead to incontinence. Urine may be retained in the bladder and then overflow past the blockage caused by the prostate. The patient has no control over this 'overflow' incontinence. A failed prostatectomy operation can also lead to incontinence. Specialist surgical advice will be needed in such cases.

9. *Bladder dysfunction.* It is now known that the bladder mechanism may go wrong in a number of ways, and these can

be investigated by special X-rays and pressure measurements in the bladder. For example some incontinent patients have a large bladder which has poor muscle tone and empties spontaneously when the volume of urine reaches a certain amount. Others have a small but 'irritable' bladder which empties small quantities of urine with no warning. These and other related forms of incontinence are not uncommon, but they are not due to dementia. They require special investigation at an incontinence clinic.

10. *The incontinence of dementia.* In the true neurological incontinence of dementia the patient has a normal bladder but the inhibitory messages from the brain are not being despatched from the frontal lobes. (In disease or injury of the spinal cord these messages are interrupted on their way to the bladder and incontinence also results.) The patient's bladder opens when it reaches a certain size and pressure. The messages *to* the brain telling of the bladder pressure and of urination may also be appreciated less and the patient is completely unaware of the problem. At early stages, however, some awareness is present and the patient may react with embarrassment, or by attempts to hide wet underclothes.

Management

As with all the other forms of disinhibition, we should search first for remediable causes or exacerbating factors.

Retraining can be very useful if the incontinence of dementia is of recent onset, giving regular reminders to the patient that she may need the toilet and praise for success. Criticism of failure is more likely to cause incontinence than cure it. Regular toileting at 2-hourly or 1-hourly intervals can help reinstitute continence, once again calm and praise being used to reinforce success. Like external controls in social disinhibition (p. 145) this technique provides a message from outside ('it is time to urinate') that previously came from inside.

Eventually, most dementia sufferers lose urinary continence for good, and require incontinence aids.

Drugs such as emepronium can inhibit the reflex to urinate and may be used to treat this type of incontinence at the early stages, but they are not always successful, and not likely to be permanently successful.

Incontinence aids of many types are available. Special absorbent pads or pants can be useful for both urinary and faecal incontinence. Protective bedding can reduce the discomfort, smell and damage of incontinence. Incontinent laundry services provide regular fresh sheets. Occasionally an in-dwelling catheter may be necessary and tolerated by the patient.

Faecal incontinence

Even more than is the case with urinary incontinence, faecal incontinence early in dementia can be taken as a sign of a separate disorder, not a consequence of the dementia. The common causes are:

1. *Constipation*. When there is a blockage in the rectum or higher up in the intestine, the movement of food becoming faecal waste continues and may overflow past the blockage. The result is foul smelling, poorly formed incontinent faeces. Relief of the constipation will cure the problem. But if the constipation has been a problem for some time, retraining of the bowel will not be immediately effective.

2. *Laxatives*. Overuse of laxatives can produce incontinence. Some patients are dependent on laxatives, and may even take them secretly, but usually this cause is easily found and corrected.

3. *Bowel diseases*. Food poisoning and other infections which cause diarrhoea, diverticular disease and less common illnesses, including ulcerative colitis and cancer of the bowel, may all lead to incontinence of faeces. If constipation and laxative overuse have been ruled out as causes of the incontinence, then these causes should be considered.

Having ruled out these medical causes, the problems of self-neglect, loss of 'conscience' and inability to find or reach the toilet, should be considered. There is no medical treatment which is likely to reverse incontinence that is due to loss of control in dementia. Much depends on avoiding constipation, good diet and regular toileting. Incontinence like this should occur late in the disease, but can still be very distressing to the patient. Prompt cleaning and changing are the best service that can be given.

Incontinence of either urine or faeces is a medical problem. It always deserves careful investigation before assuming that nothing can be done.

Fits

Fits are common in both ATD and MID. They may be caused by scarring after damage to the brain; this is certainly the case in MID. The scarring acts as a focus of irritation, and the electrical disturbances so caused lead on to a fit. There is an element of loss of control, though fits are not true disinhibitory phenomena. The fits of dementia may be of various types — focal, petit mal or grand mal.

A *focal fit* is a discharge of activity in a particular area of the cortex leading to an experience or behaviour that relates to that area (p. 88). In a fit in the motor area, specific muscles may twitch. In a temporal lobe fit, the patient may hear sounds or have other unusual experiences (called an 'aura'). Such a fit may become more generalized and turn into a grand mal fit. But *grand mal* fits can also occur without warning. These are 'major' fits, and are caused by electrical disturbances in the central parts of the brain. Because the centres which control consciousness are in the central regions (p. 49) the patient becomes unconscious during the fit while there is at the same time a generalized discharge in all areas of the brain. This leads to a contraction of all muscles (the 'tonic' phase) followed by irregular shaking of the muscles (the 'clonic' phase). After this the patient goes into a coma, a deep sleep, a confusional state or any combination of these. A *petit mal* fit is not a lesser version of a grand mal fit; it is different. There is a characteristic pattern of electrical discharge in the brain, again due to central disturbance, but the only outside evidence of the fit is a sudden and usually brief loss of consciousness or 'absence'.

If fits occur early in dementia, or repeatedly, they need investigation by a neurologist, and EEG examination to rule out other, possibly remedial, causes such as tumours. If the fits are part of the dementia, and are happening repeatedly, then an antiepileptic drug will be required.

However, the problem in dementing patients is that, although classical fits do occur, many 'turns' are not so classical and it can be difficult to be clear about what is a fit, what a dizzy turn and what a TIA.

Many severely dementing patients have repetitive twitching movements in one or a few muscles. These are called *'myoclonic jerks'*. They may respond to anti-epileptic treatment although they are not true fits.

CONCLUSION

Table 5.3 summarizes the principles that we have seen to be useful in dealing with various types of loss of control in dementia. These are all problems which cause great distress to families and staff, and sometimes to the patient herself. They are what makes a dementing patient 'psychiatric'. If they can be relieved, then the course of dementia can be smoother and less stressful.

Table 5.3 Disinhibition and its management

Steps in assessment	Management
Look for other causes of the problem	Treat cause
Examine attitudes to 'problem'	Discuss among staff and family
Look at external controls	Are these being under- or over-used
Identify circumstances of behaviour	Modify if necessary
Identify reactions of others to behaviour	Modify if necessary
Look at circumstances of 'normal' behaviour and reactions to it	Encourage this behaviour
Check that improvements are maintained	Reinforce improvement
Assess whether these techniques have worked or whether behaviour is too disturbed	Drug treatment if necessary

6

The experience of dementia

We can now understand the main changes that happen during the course of dementia, the losses and the new behaviour. They are directly caused by damage to the organic structure of the brain. The function of the damaged parts declines and consequently the patient changes. But these changes are happening to a person who lives through the experience of dementia and reacts to it, though since experience and reaction are also functions of the brain, these too will be modified and declining. In this chapter, we will see how the patient's reactions to the experience of dementia can pose problems both for herself and for others. We will also look at how to manage the distressing aspects of these reactions.

Severe dementia

What is it like to suffer from dementia? How do patients feel about the experience? To some extent these are unanswerable questions. If we take a severely demented lady, who is apparently unable to understand, who shows no evidence of any thoughts or feelings, and who is unable to speak, we can have little idea of what she is experiencing. Anything which she does experience will be quickly forgotten, and she will be unable to give a coherent account of it even to herself.

156

A fragmentary world

It is most unlikely that such a patient is 'locked in' with lots of thoughts and feelings that she cannot express, as can happen to people who suffer severe speech disorders, or severe parkinsonism. It is much more likely that there is very little mental activity at all and that she is living in a world of fragmented experience, a world of meaningless sights, sounds, smells, tastes and bodily sensations, partly experienced consciously, and unconnected to her equally fragmented emotions and actions.

We can have little conception of what these fragmentary sensation or thoughts are like, or what a fragmentary emotion is. We may be able to recognize in ourselves the experience of half-remembered ideas, of half-understood perceptions, of fleeting emotions, or vague motivations, but we experience these from a normal base. When fully conscious, our minds also contain other, more coherent ideas, our sense of self and the world around is clear, and we see these fragments as on the verge of our experience. What, however, if these were the *only* things in our minds and if that sense of 'I' was incomplete too? Would it be like the bits and pieces of experience that go through our dreams? Or is it like recalling what we can of a confusional state? The answer is 'neither', because there would never be a time when we would 'wake up' to recall what we had experienced.

Objective and subjective experience

What we can be sure of, I think, is that the experience for the *onlooker* is different from the experience for the *sufferer*. The onlooker sees the decline, the emptiness of the patient's mind, her inability to do anything for herself, her disintegrating personality, and so may feel a sense of loss, of pessimism, of boredom, of degradation.

The patient herself, on the other hand, is unlikely to be aware of or feel any these changes in a coherent fashion. She will not recall all the things that she used to be able to do and so she will be unable to recognize the change in herself. She will not be able to feel the humiliation of her dependent position. She will not sense the passage of time. Or she may experience the wrong feelings, or jumbled bits and pieces of feeling, some appropriate, some not.

It is important to remind ourselves of this, when we think of the plight of the severely demented. Our feelings about what is good or humane for a very severely demented patient cannot come from an understanding of what she feels as an individual, or of what she 'wants'. These concepts are meaningless and so any real understanding is impossible.

Respect for the severely demented

We could conclude that it does not therefore matter what we *do* to a severe dementia sufferer, for she will not understand or react. This is tempting, but it is not humane, and denies the right of the individual to reasonable care and attention when she is ill. We should instead realize that her position of helplessness demands that we pay *special* attention to her needs and treatment. It requires of us a dignified, humane approach to the dementing person, which can be difficult to sustain. This special attention is not so vital for the non-demented, for they can usually answer back, can feel offended or grateful, and can remember who is treating them well and who is treating them badly.

The 'second childhood'

Nor is it the case that the life of a very demented lady is just like that of an infant. It is true that an infant is likely to experience both the world around and its own mental content in an incomplete way. But even at early stages there is some structure and pattern to the way an infant begins to understand, feel and express itself. Despite Ribot's law, the breakdown of the mind in dementia does not exactly reverse that sequence of development. So trying to make sense of the utterances or expressions of the victim of severe dementia is unlikely to be successful. These are the random, often inappropriate, expressions of a disintegrating mind, not the half-formed products of a developing mind which will later become more organized.

Milder dementia

Just because it is impossible to understand the experience of *severe* dementia, however, we should not give up trying to understand the earlier stages. It is true that the further the process of dementia continues and the more distant from her normal experience the person becomes, the less we can comprehend of what she feels. But we can try to understand bits of her experience. Much of our understanding comes from other illness, such as strokes, which may damage brain functions partially, leaving unchanged the patient's intellect and her ability to react emotionally. In addition, although the dementia victim may not be able to tell us *all* her experiences, many early sufferers who have good insight into what is happening can describe their feelings very well. From this evidence we can try piece together a picture of what it feels like to be dementing.

The value of understanding reactions

What value will this picture serve? It is, of course, humane to try to empathize with people who are ill. If we do not empathize, we distance ourselves from them and are in danger of seeing them as things and not as people. But there are more practical reasons for wanting to understand the experience of dementia. We would, after all, expect sufferers to be horrified, to feel hopeless, depressed and anxious about the future. They need understanding and practical help to cope with these feelings.

But they sometimes appear to have no reaction at all or react only partially. Furthermore, some react in ways which we would not expect, such as by hoarding money for security, by blaming neighbours for mistakes they have made themselves, by becoming aggressive when frustrated or put under pressure, by pretending that they are perfectly well.

These reactions may puzzle us. We do not know how to respond. If we could understand *why* they were happening, we might respond more appropriately and devise treatments which could help the patient. Life might then be more tolerable both for the patient herself and for her supporters.

FACTORS AFFECTING REACTIONS TO DEMENTIA

To move from *guessing* what we would *expect* the patient to feel, to *understanding* what she *does* feel, we need to consider several factors (Fig. 6.1)

1. Her personality before the illness developed.
2. Her expectations of dementia.
3. Her insight into what is happening.
4. The changes in her personality and reactions brought about by the dementia.

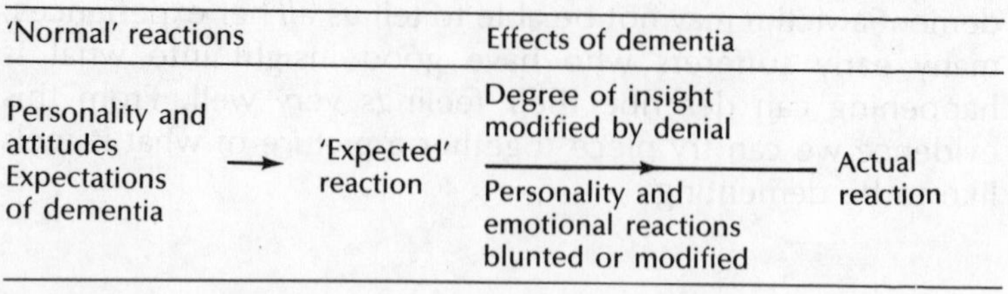

'Normal' reactions		Effects of dementia	
Personality and attitudes Expectations of dementia	→ 'Expected' reaction	Degree of insight modified by denial ──────────► Personality and emotional reactions blunted or modified	Actual reaction

Fig. 6.1 Factors affecting reactions to dementia

Personality

In Chapter 4 we saw that individual patients retain many of their personal characteristics a long way into dementia, even if these are eventually lost. If we can describe the patient's *lifelong* personality we will therefore understand many of her reactions to the illness, especially in the earlier stages.

'Personality' and *'Personality disorder'*. There is no exact science of personality. Psychologists argue about whether we can define it at all, or whether it is just a ragbag of habitual ways of behaving, which could easily be modified by changes in circumstances. And attempts to define particular personalities have varied from the description of broad types (e.g. extraverts and introverts) to a more individual description of personality 'traits'. In psychiatry, categories of 'personality disorder' are described. But it is quite difficult to say what is a 'normal' personality and what is abnormal or disordered.

To avoid some of these critisisms it is best to take a position that is not too dogmatic. There *are* some characteristic patterns in the way people behave, in how people deal with crises, in their ways of relating to others, and in their attitudes and interests. These can be roughly described and categorized as different personality *types*, but such descriptions are not very reliable. Sometimes a person may wish that her own personality type were different, or other people may complain about it. She can be said to have a personality problem or disorder. Let us look at how people of different personality types are likely to react to dementia.

Types of personality and their reactions to dementia

Extraverts and Introverts. People who are extraverted and sociable often cope quite well with dementia. If they keep their personality they are popular patients and they accept help cheerfully. On the other hand, people who are introverted or *schizoid* (detached and emotionally cold), while they may not mind the isolation of old age, being usually quite self-sufficient, often dislike the communal aspects of care, such as going to a day hospital, or living in a home with a group of other people. It is unfortunate for such people that so many services are organized on group lines.

Dependent personality. Some people look at the world as if they could not achieve much by themselves; they feel the need of someone or something as a crutch; they may actually be quite capable of coping but feel that they cannot. We might expect such people to adjust well to dementia, because they will accept the need for outside help readily. They tend to ask for services, sometimes even ending up with too much help. On the other hand they may be reluctant to show initiative or to keep active and independent with their remaining faculties. We may have to spend time encouraging these 'dependent' people that they can cope alone, or do more for themselves.

Independent personality. Others are of more independent type and they dislike relying on others. They will resist the increasing dependence of dementia, even when they actually do not have the capacity to cope. Thus they often make 'bad' patients, since they may refuse the help that family and others offer. They may even end up requiring compulsory measures to ensure that they get help (Ch. 9). They are 'good' patients, however, if independence is needed. So they may do well in retraining programmes, though they will be impatient with their helpers and sometimes unrealistically hopeful about coping.

Basically, such people need to feel that they are in charge of their own destiny and that they will 'die with their boots on'. So an 'infantilizing' or patronizing approach will not work with them. Family and staff should contrive to let the patient feel that *she* is making the decision, even though that is something of a white lie. She is likely to protest strongly when help is introduced without her full agreement or when she has to move into care. But in fact it is remarkable how often that protest is short-lived, for secretly she appreciates the more dependent position.

Paranoid personality. The paranoid person tends to be suspicious or critical of the outside world, especially when anything goes wrong. Such a person is often also extremely independent-minded. When dementia occurs, she may blame others when *she* makes mistakes and may be suspicious of the motives behind offers of help. This type of reaction is discussed further on page 181.

Obsessional personality. The person who is orderly, punctual or rather rigid by nature, or the person who is prone to recurrent self-doubts and who needs to check repeatedly that everything around her is exactly right will find the experience of dementia distressing, for she is faced with a disintegration of order, forgetfulness of time, loss of control and lowering of standards. And the changes brought about in her personality due to the dementia are likely to be very obvious to her family. For both these reasons obsessional people tend to be referred for help very early in dementia.

Hysterical personality. A person who tends to live on the surface of things, dramatizing little problems, needing the attention of others to feel good herself, perhaps playing people off against each other, but forming few deep relationships, is said to have a hysterical personality type. Faced with the multiple problems of dementia she may in fact cope surprisingly well. But sometimes such a patient will behave in a more typical demanding way, acting 'iller' then she actually is. There is always the danger that real illness or distress is overlooked, that she cries 'wolf' too often. Such a patient requires the same attention as others, no more and no less, but working out her *actual* needs can be difficult.

Psychopathic personality. The psychopath is concerned only with her own immediate needs. She is impulsive and demanding, uses people without concern for their needs, and may be aggressive or even criminal without conscience. Many psychopaths seem to 'cool down' in old age, so psychopathy is not a major problem among dementia sufferers, but one or two can add to the management problems of a ward or a home.

'Normal' personality. There is no such thing as a normal reaction to dementia, for there is really no such thing as a normal personality type. Most individuals have little bits of one or more of the above personality traits within them, though some are classics of a particular type. Each person deserves to be understood as an individual.

Expectations of dementia

If asked how common 'confusion' is among elderly people, both young and old people regularly overestimate, some guessing at a figure as high as 50% rather than the true figure of no more than one in ten. Those who work in the health or social services are particularly likely to overestimate because, as mentioned in Chapter 3, they see a concentration of dementing people in their care. But the tendency is probably part of that general set of negative attitudes to old age which has been called 'ageism'. The corollary of this sort of belief is that people who are not demented in old age are treated as remarkable, particularly if they remain active, socially involved and able to keep up to date ('She actually still goes to the bingo at 85!')

So, many people must expect that they will suffer some degree of dementia. Some of these people will know something of what dementia is like, but others will have a more or less distorted or imcomplete view. Everybody knows that *memory* is lost in 'confusion' or dementia. Many indeed seem to believe that *all* old people lose their memories. But not many realize that true dementia involves the mutiple losses described in Chapter 4. And there is a tendency to think of two conditions, one a mild memory impairment which is not a causes for concern, the other severe dementia, needing total care. The evidence suggests that this is not a proper distinction and that, unless some other cause is found, a person with mild impairment will, in time, become more severely impaired.

Those who think that many or all old people suffer some sort of relatively mild memory impairment are quite prepared for the early changes of dementia. When their memory begins to fail they are likely to say that they expected this, that it is a normal part of old age and that, therefore, there is little to worry about. They are apt to ignore the other evidence of their decline and eventually to play down the degree of their memory impairment. They continue to claim to be happy and see little need for help or care.

Experience in the family

Previous experience colours our expectations. Dementia is a common condition, so many people have at least a little exposure to it. If one member of a family develops dementia the other family members are likely to have a horror of developing it too and will fear particular behaviour problems which affected their relative, such as wandering or disinhibited behaviour. If the relative got unsatisfactory care, then family members may assume that all care is like that. They will of course be recalling mainly the 'outside' of the relative's dementia (p. 156) rather than thinking what the experience was like for the sufferer herself.

Huntington's chorea. The family will worry even more if they consider genetic factors. In Huntington's chorea families, this worry becomes a realistic fear since the child of an affected parent has a 50% chance of developing the condition (Fig. 6.2) and *each* child of the afffected parent that is born has the same 50% risk — the risk does not reduce when an older brother or sister possesses the gene. This is a frightening prospect for each child, but they are in a still greater dilemma. The parent may develop the illness relatively early in life, even in their 30s, but it may be later, in their 50s or 60s or rarely even later that it begins. So the children may not know until they are adults themselves whether they are at risk or not. When they come to think of producing the next

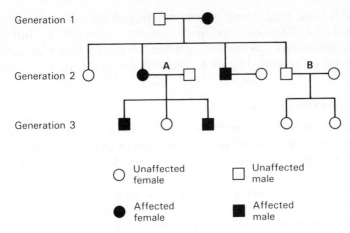

Fig. 6.2 A typical family pedigree of Huntington's chorea. There is a 50% chance at each birth that couple A will produce an affected child. None of couple B's children will be affected. However, those in Generation 2 are unlikely to know whether they are in category A or category B until after they have had their families.

generation, the grandchildren, they may not know if they are passing on a 50% chance or no chance at all.

Genetic counselling services can help prospective parents come to a decision, but with such a wide variation in the risks and possibilities it must remain up to the prospective parent to make the final decision. The situation is made more difficult by the tendency of some Huntington's chorea families to conceal the illness from the next generation, making proper genetic counselling impossible, but more enlightened attitudes are gaining ground.

Recent developments in 'gene-mapping' and 'genetic markers' will eventually allow much more exact genetic counselling. Diagnosis before birth, and therapeutic abortion could also be a possibility. Unfortunately these tests are not yet 100% accurate. And although there will be enormous relief for those who can be told that they do not have the gene, will not suffer the illness, and will not pass it to their children, the consequences of telling someone that they do carry the gene could be tragic, since there is as yet no treatment.

ATD and MID. There is not enough genetic risk in the other forms of dementia to merit genetic counselling, but in Alzheimer-type dementia, families of sufferers are at some increased risk (p. 19), so a little worry is justified.

False expectations

All this expectation and worry is excessive and in some sense unnecessary. No individual can predict that they will suffer ATD or MID. They cannot predict how dementia will change them if they do develop it, what symptoms they will show and what help they will need. And their ideas of how they would react reflect more on their current state than on what their *actual* experience of dementia will be years later. Just as a child may swear that she will never marry, yet 20 years later is married and happily settled, so we look forward to old age and see its horrors as if we would experience them as we are now, not as we will be then.

People anticipating dementia may see it as a bleak, hopeless, dependent existence compared to their present active lives. They do not see the greater acceptance of old age, the blunting effects of dementia and the effects of loss of insight and memory on the sufferer's experience. So young people thinking of dementia anticipate that they would become severely depressed if they developed it, or even that they would commit suicide. Yet the suicide rate is actually remarkably low and even depression is not universal by any means.

More realistically, younger people see the burden that dementia is to the rest of a family and so think that they would inevitably need to be in institutional care. If they have negative views of care, then the outlook can seem bleak indeed.

People who are frightened by the prospect of dementia may react badly if they see evidence of its beginnings. They may imagine it is developing when they are in fact well; they may try to hide it if it does develop, or become very distressed.

Preparing for dementia

The family. Since there are such varied and sometimes

inaccurate attitudes to dementia, there is a major need to educate the public, and particularly the families of dementing patients. People in general need more facts about the likelihood of any individual developing dementia, about what the illness is like, and what can be done to help. Families should be told, if they ask, about the slightly increased genetic risk, but should be reassured that the risk is still small and that there are plenty of other commoner conditions, such as heart disease, which are more likely to kill them. It is not unreasonable for families to discuss among themselves what help would be available from each other if it were ever needed.

The individual. An older person worried by the prospect of dementia, or indeed any disablement, can be helped if they have comtemplated the worst and been reassured that reasonable amounts of family support would be at hand. They will not, however, be helped if the reassurance is false or if they try to demand impossible support or to close options. 'If I get confused, you must never put me in a home' or 'You'll look after me, won't you?' merely store up difficulties for the future. Dementia is also an important subject for discussion in retirement courses and day centres. It should not be brushed under the carpet.

The subject should be raised particularly when an elderly person is planning a change in her living circumstances, to move in with her younger family, or go to sheltered housing. The onset of dementia after she has moved can be disastrous, but it is worse if the patient has been misled into thinking that her place in the home is permanent no matter what happens. There *are* circumstances where families or sheltered housing schemes cannot cope. It may seem harsh to bring up the subject of an illness which only affects a minority of people. But the fact that it *has* been broached and that no unrealistic expectations have been raised, can lessen the person's feeling of rejection if help has to be called in later, or she has to move to a more sheltered environment.

Insight

We have seen that patients come to dementia with differing personality attributes and differing expectations, attitudes and experience, and that these will influence their individual reactions to the illness. But how strong and how appropriate their reactions are depend also on how much they understand of what is going on — their *insight*. Insight can be described as the awareness by a patient that she has changed and that the changes are due to an illness, in other words, the awareness that she is dementing. It also implies knowing the extent and severity of the illness. It does *not* mean knowing all about the workings of the brain or the chemistry of Alzheimer-type dementia. It refers to ordinary personal experience and understanding.

At its simplest we can see that a person who realizes that she is suffering from dementia, who is aware that she is making mistakes of memory, not looking after herself properly etc., will react in a very different way from a person who is showing the same decline but is totally unaware that anything is wrong. But insight is a very complicated concept and it is difficult to be exact about it.

Stages of insight

A number of stages are involved. Let us consider a previously well-organized lady who is forgetting to light her gas fire when she puts it on, forgetting to collect her pension, or forgetting appointments. There has been a slow decline in her general ability to look after herself, and to an outsider, it is clear that she is beginning to suffer dementia. In order to realize this herself she needs first to realize that she has made these mistakes. She may not recall them, or even seem unaware of the mistakes at the time they occurred (see p. 93). Even if she recognizes and recalls her mistakes she must also be able to remember her *normal* way of behaving and make the logical connection that there has been a change. Her ability to think logically as well as her ability to remember may be impaired. The frontal lobe functions of conscience and judgement are needed for her to show concern about the mistakes she is making. So, even before we consider how she might react to her insight, there are many reasons why insight may be imperfect or even absent. Furthermore, the decline in insight may begin very early on in the illness.

Denial of insight

We have already noted the tendency for patients to assume, even if they have some insight, that their impairments are minor and an ordinary part of old age. Some of this is due to ignorance. Some is due to *denial*. Denial is a common defence mechanism which people employ to shield themselves from some unpleasant truth. They act as if it were not true. This self-deception or deception of others could be considered as dishonest, but as we will see, it is a normal part of the universal grief reaction to any loss (p. 190), 'It hasn't happened' protecting against the full flood of distress that might be paralysing. Dementia is both an unpleasant truth and a loss. Not only are the person's mental faculties being lost, but independence and eventually life itself are lost. It is not surprising, then, that many sufferers shield themselves against full awareness of their decline and fate.

We can be sure that patients deny their insight, at least to other people. Some patients admit their insight to one person and not to another. Others will deny insight at the beginning of a conversation, but later, when they feel more secure, acknowledge that they do understand their position. The lady who hides her wet knickers is aware that she has been incontinent; she is not denying the fact to herself, but is trying to deny it to others. She is protecting herself against the ridicule and rejection which she may quite understandably expect.

But we can guess that many even deny the facts to themselves. They seem totally aware of their memory impairment but deny the consequences. They may have the evidence of a burnt pan or a neglected house in front of them and blatantly deny that the evidence exists or has anything to do with them. Both true lack of insight, due to agnosia or other impairments, and denial are involved in this reaction, though it is difficult to know in what proportions.

Estimating denial. Estimating the extent to which denial makes the patient play down her reactions either to herself or to others cannot therefore be more than guesswork. It is usually a mistake to accuse patients of 'pretending' that they are not ill. For denial is an important defence, Attacking defences usually makes a person defend herself more rather than less; attacking defences, which *we* imagine are present but which do not exist, is wrong.

Estimating insight

Insight, then, is a difficult concept to pin down and may be hidden by denial. In practice, the main evidence we can obtain about how much a patient knows of her illness is from her reactions to it. We would expect someone who had a fairly general understanding of dementia to react with distress. It would be like mourning a loss (p. 189). It would be a shock at first, then depressing or anxiety-provoking, and she would be forced to reconsider all her plans for the future, her relationships with others, her ability to be independent. In a way she would be preparing for her own death. She would also understand fully why other people are reacting to her differently.

As we shall see, patients' actual reactions are usually much less dramatic and far-reaching than this, though a partial grief reaction is quite common. So we must conclude that, even allowing for some denial , insight is probably limited in most people.

On the other hand, the patient who totally lacks insight is likely to be happy with herself, not realizing that anything is wrong, but completely baffled by the reactions of others. Family and strangers suggest a need for help, even that she should leave her own home, but she can see no need for any change at all. The majority of sufferers fall somewhere between these two extremes of total insight and total lack of insight.

'Treating' lack of insight

Should we try to improve insight? In theory it would seem better that patients with any sort of illness should know that they are ill and learn something of the nature of their illness. This would help them to co-operate in a treatment programme, and to report changes in their condition. And so it is with dementia. The lady who has complete insight is likely to be co-operative in care, wish to do whatever will improve the quality of her life and wish to avoid being a burden on others. The lady with no insight will have difficulty with co-operation, will resent intrusions in her life and see no reason for outside help. So it is reasonable to try to improve insight. This can be done· by reminding the patient of the evidence of her failing abilities, explaining how dementia progresses and showing that she will therefore need gradually increasing help.

But this will not always work or may work only partially. For the patient may be *incapable* of proper insight because of her dementia. Or she may have chosen to deny insight and find moving from that position unthinkable. And in many cases insight may actually cause distress. The patient may react angrily, dismissing what is said as nonsense, or she may see the tragedy of her position and be very upset. All these are reasons for being extremely sensitive when trying to improve insight. It can be done to a certain extent, it can be helpful, but it can be distressing. It is not always the right thing to do.

Mistaken insight

Finally we should not forget that group of people who have *mistaken* insight, who believe that they are suffering from dementia, but in fact are well. These include the people mentioned in Chapter 2, who suffer from acute confusion, physical illnesses or pseudodementia, and who imagine that their memory losses are permanent, as well as the ordinary old people who believe that the ordinary changes of ageing are the beginnings of dementia (p. 39). Proper diagnosis and information to the elderly who are ill and general education about old age and dementia should reduce this problem.

But there are also people who are just beginning to dement and suffer great uncertainty about whether they will get worse or better. There is little that can be done at present to re-assure them. They will fear all the losses of dementia, the dependence, the disintegration of the self, the loss of control, the burden on others. These fears are powerful and difficult to cope with. They need the promise of diagnosis as soon as possible, a check for remediable causes of their mild memory loss and honest reassurance about what help would be available if they were to go on to suffer more severe dementia.

Personality changes in dementia

We might now expect to be able to understand the individual reactions of patients to their dementia. But there is a further complication. For the person who is experiencing the dementia is being changed in herself *by* the dementia. So it is not the old personality with old expectations who is reacting to the illness, but a shrunken or modified personality with less understanding or mistaken ideas. Her actual reaction will be a mixture of some bits of her old ways of reacting and some bits of new ways.

Normal changes of old age

Indeed, even before the dementia begins, an older person's personality may have changed a little with age. There are enormous variations between people in how much of a change this is, but there are some general trends, which have already been mentioned (p. 36). Slowness, cautiousness, rigidity, dislike of change or newness, more emotional detachment and a tendency to withdraw from involvement with activities or peoople all occur to a greater or lesser extent in older people. In terms of our list of personality types (p. 161), people become a little more introverted and obsessional.

Effects on reactions. The reactions we expect from a dementia sufferer will be modified by these changes. An older patient may not only expect dementia to happen as part of old age, but may react less emotionally, and keep her feelings to herself rather than discussing them with others. She may try stoically to keep to a routine, unexciting way of life. She may react badly to sudden changes, sudden new faces, and be less inclined to mix with others than might have been the case in her earlier years. As with other older people we may feel that just a little change, such as joining a lunch club or taking up a hobby, would help matters enormously. But her rigidity, cautiousness and social withdrawal get in the way. These changes occur less in younger, 'pre-senile' patients.

Effects of changes due to dementia

Decline in personality. Chapter 4 and 5 have included many examples of how dementia affects personality and emotional reactions, by causing either a decline or a change. The decline in positive personality features and in emotional life means that most people react much more blandly to their dementia than we might expect. They are a 'shadow of their former selves'. But, as with everything else in dementia, the decline is gradual, and at the beginning of the process, the personality is largely intact. This explains the paradox that the *patients' reactions tend to be more of a problem in earlier, milder dementia than they are at later, more severe stages.* In severe dementia, when the emotions and personality are destroyed, the patient is unable to react at all.

Changed personality. If the patient's personality changes because of the development of emotional lability, or because of the appearance of a completely new trait such as demandingness, obsessionality, irritability, or paranoia, then we must expect completely new types of reaction. For relatives, this is one of the most distressing facets of dementia — the patient reacts like a 'stranger'. And when decline and disinhibition get mixed together the reactions become a jumble. Once again, the tendency to show 'new' personality features is greatest early in dementia (p. 138). So these new and complicated reactions are most likely in mild cases.

Preserved personality. It should be recalled, however, that some patients, especially those with patchy damage in multi-infarct dementia, may retain many of their old personality traits until quite late in the illness. Even here the general tendency to be more rigid and to give stereotyped responses can mean that the patient's reactions become a sort of exaggerated caricature of her previous self. It is sometimes said that in old age our worst personality characteristics become exaggerated and 'stuck'. If there is any truth in that it is even more true among sufferers from dementia.

Whether exaggerated or not, the fact that personality is often retained in MID means that these patients tend to show more reaction to their dementia, and that their reactions are more understandable. In ATD, on the other hand, it is often the case that insight declines at roughly the same rate as everything else. The result may be a vague, ill-formed regret or seeming indifference to the illness. This relative lack of reaction can be frustrating for relatives, but a blessing for the patient who accepts her declining abilities with a smile.

Conclusion

Despite all these modifications it is still possible in many cases to explain and understand how the individual sufferer reacts to her dementia. It is certainly very worthwhile *trying* to understand, using information about her previous personality, her expectations and experience and the changes in her personality with age and dementia. For if we understand we can empathize and if we empathize we will see ways of helping her cope better.

TYPES OF REACTION

We will now examine some of the particular ways in which patients react to the various symptoms of dementia. Obviously one person may react differently to different symptoms. For example, since memory impairment tends to be expected, many sufferers are remarkably sanguine about its appearance and effects (if they can remember them!). On the other hand, dressing dyspraxia, which is not expected, is much more distressing. So *expectations* are important.

But it is also *easier* for a patient to be aware of some types of symptom than of others. The best example relates to the two main types of dysphasia seen particularly in stroke patients. When there is a *receptive* dysphasia (p. 94) the patient has difficulty in understanding the meaning of words, her own as well as others. The result is not only that she may fail to understand what is said to her but that, when she responds with meaningless words, she does not realize what she is doing and so is not distressed by her mistakes. In *expressive* dysphasia (p. 114) on the other hand, if reception is good, the patient is painfully aware of the mistakes she is making and is likely to feel frustrated and distressed.

Depression

Grief

Depression (Table 6.1) is the most understandable reaction to the multiple losses of dementia. It is the central emotion in the *grief reaction*, a general human response to a loss of any kind. Grief reactions will be discussed more fully in Chapter 7, when we consider how families react, for the losses of dementia are usually felt much more by relatives and friends than by the patient herself. Not only is she likely to have limited awareness of her symptoms, but she may have only a patchy recollection of her normal self to compare with. If she cannot see any loss, she will not become depressed. However, in the early stages, those with good insight will be all too aware of their losses and will react more appropriately.

Just as with other depressed people, a patient who is depressed because of dementia needs the chance to talk about her feelings of loss to someone whom she respects and trusts. She can feel reassured and supported by knowing that

Table 6.1 Depression and dementia

Cause of depression	Management
Reaction to losses and changed circumstances	Guide through stages of mourning Adjust circumstances Reassuring, empathic, non-critical response
Chronic reactive depression	Antidepressants if managements above have failed
Disinhibited depression	Examine and adjust circumstances and consequences Tranquillizer or antidepressant
Depressive illness	Antidepressants
Depressive illness with pseudo-dementia	After antidepressant treatment, re-check evidence of dementia
Apathy due to organic damage	Social stimulation Try antidepressants
'Face to the wall' phenomenon	Look for causes — physical illness, depression, drugs, organic apathy

someone understands, even if she does not quite grasp all that is said, or quickly forgets it.

Recovery

Recovering from a grief reaction, however, requires an eventual move from feeling and talking to a stage of planning and doing. For the best outcome will occur if the sufferer can make changes in her life which help her adjust to her new situation. This is the recovery phase of mourning (p. 188). It can be an almost impossible task for a dementing person on her own, since it requires changing attitudes, changing relationships, changing activities. She will find all these changes difficult to contemplate, never mind carry out.

Helping recovery. If we are to help the patient recover her self-esteem and feeling of well-being we need to look more closely at the causes of her depression. Often she will be more distressed by the *circumstances* she is facing (increasing dependence) than by her actual symptoms (memory impairment, dysphasis etc.). If this is the case then there may be quite a lot of adjustment which can be made to help her. The classic example is of the lady who has to lose her independence by going to a residential home. She will mourn her loss of independence. But she can get through her depression and feel better again if she adjusts to life in the home — if she 'makes the best of it'. She must learn how to live with other residents and staff, adjust to different rules and routines, and learn to get satisfaction from different activities than those that gave her satisfaction in her own home.

If she were not dementing we could hope that she would make these changes herself. But in dementia, family and staff will likely have to make some of the adjustments for her, changing the subject away from her depressing thoughts of loss, and steering her quite actively into new interests and relationships. It is perfectly reasonable to exert pressure like this, if the alternative is that she will never get out of her depression.

Sometimes a patient feels depressed by thinking that her symptoms are affecting others. It may be that, rightly or wrongly, she feels rejected by the family because of her poor communication, or an embarrassing decline in her habits. Or maybe she feels that she is left out of decisions and that her choices are made for her. Or that she is disliked by staff. All these feelings lead to lowering of self-esteem and depression. Reassurance may help, but a change of attitude on the part of the *other* people involved, giving her more positive support, allowing her more say, showing that she is appreciated despite her disabilities, may be most reassuring of all, and so help recovery.

Chronic depression

Some patients will manage to reach or even get through the recovery phase. Others do not and become chronically depressed. In many cases it will be difficult to tell the difference between this state of chronic depressive *feelings* as a reaction to dementia, and the state of chronic 'stuck' depressive *expression* due to disinhibition (p. 137). But, whichever the cause, the gradual decline in all aspects of emotional life in dementia will eventually lead to the disappearance of these chronic depressive states. While the depression lasts, however, it is reasonable to try treatment with a full course of antidepressant drugs.

Depressive illness

True depressive illness — that is, depression which is not readily understandable (p. 57), and which may be part of a long-standing recurrent depressive or manic-depressive illness — can occur during a dementia, and will require its standard treatment with antidepressant drugs or ECT. In the later stages of dementia, this sort of depression may only be discernible by its physical symptoms, since the patient cannot explain how she feels. There will be loss of appetite, slowing of actions, a downcast look, perhaps a worsening in the mornings. The patient may be thought to have 'turned her face to the wall'. But the past history of previous depressions gives the clue that this episode should be treated and the patient may then return to her previous happy, though demented, state.

'Face to the wall'

'Turning the face to the wall' is an apparently voluntary desire
to die , expressed usually by withdrawal, apathy and refusal
to eat or drink. It must be distinguished not only from depressive illness, but from physical illness and the effects of drugs
— for it would be wrong to miss these (Table 6.1). But that
being said, we must assume that some dementing patients
choose this variant of suicide. It sometimes *appears* to
happen in very severely demented people, but they are
unlikely to have enough understanding to make such a logical
decision. It may then represent a severe decline in motivation
due to brain damage rather than a logical reaction to the
dementia. True reactive depression and a consequent 'wish
to die' are more likely to occur in mildly dementing patients
who also have physical disabilities and who have some insight
into their condition.

More active intentions of suicide are rare in dementia but
not uncommon in those who fear dementia, e.g. the relatives
of Huntington's chorea patients, or those who *think* they
suffer it but do not, e.g. sufferers from the pseudodementia
of depression.

Anxieties and fears

Anxiety is again an understandable emotion. The patient is
entering an unknown world. It is reasonable that she should
be apprehensive about what will happen to her and the
changes that will come in her life.

She may have one or several specific fears — fear of missing
appointments, fear of losing her keys, or losing her money,
fear of getting lost outside. Or she may be anxious about her
relatives' attitudes. She may worry that she will do embarrassing things in public, or that she will lose control of
herself. She may even see a glimpse of the loss of her personality and identity which will occur later in dementia, and be
terrified.

Expressions of anxiety. Anxiety may be expressed directly
or indirectly. She may be able to talk about her fears, but if
she is unwilling to talk, or can no longer communicate, then

all that we can observe is restlessness (Table 5.2) or the physical expressions of anxiety such as tremor, sweating and a rapid pulse. We then have to guess what is causing her anxiety and what will help. Much of the restlessness that occurs in dementia is probably due to anxiety, particularly fear of being lost and anxiety about forgetfulness.

Reactions to anxiety. The patient may try to do things to relieve her own anxiety. Writing down reminders on slips of paper, asking the time, asking the family for reassurance — all are typical. But each has its problems. Reminders get lost or are illegible, causing even greater anxiety. Long-suffering neighbours are knocked up repeatedly by night and by day to be asked the time. The family get infuriated with repetitive calls for reassurance and begin to feel antagonistic towards the patient. Indeed, this repetitive questioning is one of the most difficult things for relatives to tolerate. It is made worse when the patient seems quite egocentric and oblivious of the distress she is causing. It is no wonder that some patients end up trying to avoid embarrassment and hostile reactions by social withdrawal (p. 182).

Management of anxiety

Listening and reassurance. We cannot stop anxious patients from trying to relieve their anxieties by themselves, but it is often better if they talk over their anxieties with others. Discussing the reality of the situation is helpful, for some fears are groundless and reassurance can easily be given. The problem in listening to and reassuring a dementing person is that she may forget that she has been reassured and return with the same anxiety again and again. Eventually, the long-suffering listener must decide whether there is any real purpose being served or whether the request for reassurance has merely become a habit which is being *encouraged* by the reassurance and is leading nowhere (p. 146). Reassurance will certainly not help if the 'anxiety' is not a reaction to the uncertainty of her circumstances, but is either a manifestation of physical discomfort, a disinhibited emotion, or part of a depressive illness.

Relieving tension. Reducing anxiety by techniques such as

relaxation exercises or breathing exercises are quite often only a limited help to an anxious dementing patient because these techniques require sustained effort and learning. Other people have to help her relax by using a calm tone of voice, a gentle approach, soothing touch, music or relaxing activity.

Removing causes of anxiety. Taking pressure off the patient will be helpful. If she is bombarded with problems to solve she will become more anxious. In other words, a generally less demanding environment is best. The behavioural chart approach (Table 5.1) may help, showing in what situations she is most anxious and identifying what or who is raising the tension.

Memory aids (p. 106) used judiciously can reassure the patient and prevent her from having to ask others for reassurance. Anxiety about mobility or falls may be helped by physiotherapy or walking aids (p. 120). The person who is anxious needs the reassurance that gaps in her abilities are being filled. She may even feel the need of more help than is really necessary. We may have to go along with this feeling for a while if she cannot otherwise learn to regain her self-confidence. But once she has gained confidence, the extra help can gradually be dispensed with.

Drugs. As with anti-depressants, anti-anxiety (or 'anxiolytic') drugs should only be used if anxiety is severe or 'stuck'. If they are used, it should only be for a short period. They can, however, be very helpful. A lady who is so fretful about her inability to remember things that her anxiety actually makes her memory performance worse can be helped by an anxiolytic drug to feel more at ease and so perform better. The same can apply to a patient with expressive dysphasia who gets so anxious that she speaks worse rather than better the more she tries.

Frustration

This is the feeling of a person who knows what she would like to do but cannot do it. The example of expressive dysphasia is typical (p. 116). But the same can apply to all expressive or physical activities, such as mobility, and tasks needing co-ordination, such as dressing, washing, and feeding. It can also apply to memories which 'won't come' or thoughts that 'get lost'. The expression of frustration is a plea for help. The person who is frustrated needs a realistic assessment of what her abilities are and of what she can be expected to manage. Then she needs positive help with gap filling to prevent frustration building up. Praise for small successes, and avoiding comment on failures can also encourage self- confidence.

Guilt

A sense of failure can lead on to self-blame. The patient feels that if she is not doing things right it is her own fault, or she may even blame the whole illness on herself. This feeling can be an important part of any depression, and particularly depressive illness. If it is a reaction to dementia then reassurance that her failures are not her fault, but are part of the general decline, which she cannot help, is important.

Paranoid thinking

This is, for some reasons, rather more common in dementia than guilt,or perhaps it is just more obvious. If things are going wrong the patient tends to blame others. This sort of feeling arises particularly in paranoid or independent, proud personalities, but can occur in almost any patient. If a previously houseproud dementing lady leaves a pan on the cooker and it burns, she cannot believe that it was her fault, for she will not remember doing it. She believe she could never do such a thing. So she blames the lady next door. If she cannot locate the special place where she left her money, or her underclothes, or her key, she cannot believe that she has gone to look in the wrong place and so blames her home help or begins to believe that there is an intruder.

The paranoid patient can be difficult to handle. It is important first to check whether there is any truth in her beliefs — it is, after all, not uncommon for people to steal from dementia sufferers! If there is no truth in her story, then the reality of the situation should be explained simply and calmly, and not by getting into an argument. If an argument

seems likely to develop it may be best to leave the explanations for a while, and try to change the subject, for she may
quickly forget her accusations.

Mild suspiciousness may respond to such techniques, but
the problem with paranoid thinking is that it is based on lack
of trust and so that patient finds it hard to believe in reassurance. Repeated reassuring explanations may be used as
evidence that 'something is up'. On the other hand, 'going
along with' delusions merely encourages the patient to
believe that she is right.

Drug treatment is therefore more likely to be needed for
paranoid reactions than for other reactions to dementia. The
phenothiazines and related drugs are best but there is only
a moderate chance of success.

Embarrassment

The lady who hides her wet knickers is acting out of embarrassment, the feeling that one has done something which will
be ridiculed by others. Embarrassment is felt mostly by
patients who are disinhibited but retain some insight. For
example, a patient may lose her temper over nothing and
realize how distressing this is to her family. Her embarrassment can be helped if the family reassure her that they
understand that she has difficulty controlling her feelings
because of an illness and that they are not offended by her
anger. This will also help them to avoid responding angrily
back and so worsening the situation.

Withdrawal

All these emotional reactions are distressing. It is not
surprising therefore that one of the commonest reactions to
dementia is to withdraw. This withdrawal can take many
forms. The patient may simply be quieter than usual because
of embarrassment or depression. She may drift out of her
usual social activities — church, club, family visits. At the
extreme, she may become completely isolated.

Effects of withdrawal. The dangers of this type of reaction
are, first, that she may become detached from reality, and may

be more inclined to live in her own world of long ago; second, there are physical dangers, namely self-neglect, reduced mobility, and illness due to immobility; and, third, she may get insufficient treatment for all her problems because she is not asking for help. Unfortunately, withdrawal may be quietly accepted or even encouraged by friends and relatives because *they* are embarrassed, or guilty about not helping, or feel they cannot communicate with her. Other common problems such as poor hearing, poor eyesight and poor mobility can add to her tendency to withdraw.

Stimulation. In assessing the deficits of dementia, we need to recognize that some of the patient's losses will appear worse than they actually are because of this withdrawal. The person who is beginning to have a speech problem and gets no practice at speaking is at a disadvantage. So is the person whose self-care or continence is declining and who has withdrawn so that no-one is around to stimulate her to do better. It is these patients who may respond best to gap filling and retraining. The stimulation and confidence given by company and the expectation of higher standards can encourage them to use what abilities they have more fully.

Withdrawn patients can even appear severely demented when their dementia is actually very mild. A patient who has had no stimulation and no practice of her skills for some time will 'come alive' when she moves from a neglected house into a residential home or hospital, or even when a visitor starts to visit on a regular basis. But in bringing people 'out of themselves' we should keep in mind that the withdrawal has occured for a reason, being due either to the patient's feeling of distress or to the reactions of others, and we should try to deal with that reason sensitively and actively.

Covering-up

This is a more active response to the distress of dementia than withdrawal. The patient tries to pretend that she is not dementing. The reaction is related to the defence of denial discussed earlier (p. 169). It is understandable that covering-up should happen, but it is almost impossible to discover whether it is a conscious or an unconscious action. Possibly at first there is a large conscious element, an attempt to get over the embarrassment of forgetfulness, but later some of the covering-up response seem to become automatic.

Confabulation

It is a curious fact that people whose intellectual powers are supposed to be declining can become expert at covering-up. Yet they do and can learn very effective and sophisticated ways of diverting and fooling others.

The classic response is called *confabulation*. This was in the past associated principally with Korsakoff's syndrome (p. 55), but it can in fact occur in patients who have any sort of memory impairment. When answering questions that test her memory, instead of saying that she does not know, the patient gives an answer which is a guess at what might be true, often based on her past life or habits. Her answer is usually delivered in a confident tone as if she was trying to fool the questioner. And, surprisingly, sometimes it does. But often her answer is very obviously untrue.

A more charitable explanation of confabulation suggests that it arises because memories are not stored in the correct time sequence (p. 102) and so are retrieved in the wrong order. So on old memory may be recalled in place of a recent one.

Confabulation is only one form of covering up. Table 6.2 gives a few examples of other methods. The difficulty is that all of these can work very well. The result is that family or friends may not realize how severely impaired the patient is. And professionals can be fooled too. We find that the patient has steered the conversation away from the questions we wished to ask and on to old stories or pleasantries. Interviewing may therefore involve a lot of determination to keep the patient on the track. However, we should always remember that covering up and denial occur because of distress and that uncovering can therefore lead to distress. If we need to know the facts of how seriously demented someone is, we may be forced to produce some of that distress for a brief period. But after that, there is little point unless we are sure that she will eventually be able to drop her defence and be more honest without becoming distressed.

Table 6.2 Covering-up when the honest answer is 'I don't know'

Question	Answer
'What day is it?'	'At my age you don't bother with these things.' 'You've got me at a bad time.' 'What day is it?' — asking a relative 'Let me look at my paper.' 'It's Wednesday.' — confabulation 'It's a lovely day.' — pretending to misunderstand 'Can't hear you.' 'Don't ask silly questions.' 'Do *you* not know?' 'You're asking too many questions.'

Egocentricity and altruism

For many dementia sufferers, the world contracts. Their ability to deal with others declines, they may withdraw from social contacts, and they become more egocentric. This is very distressing for relatives who get demands but no thanks from the patient. But some patients are very aware of the effects of their dementia on others and react, not with embarrassment at their condition (which is egocentric) but by trying to lighten the burden and distress that they as patients are causing. This more altruistic feeling can make a patient play down her own needs and emphasize the needs of the family for relief or support. It can be a convenient and helpful feeling but if it is excessive, her needs may be ignored. Throughout our dealings with dementia, we need to keep as balanced a view as we possibly can of the patient's actual needs, not relying only on her emotional view or our emotional view.

CONCLUSION: COPING WITH DEMENTIA

I have emphasised that all these reactions are understandable. What then is the proper reaction — what does 'coping with dementia' mean? The answer is that there is no 'proper' way, there are only multitudes of individual ways. We might say that those whose reactions cause distress to themselves or others need special help, but even where no big problems arise, *some* distress can be expected, some withdrawal from

distressing situations, some attempts to pretend that everything is normal. It would be unusual for a patient who has any
degree of insight to sail through dementia without feeling any
distress. We must be aware of that distress, and help when
necessary

7

The experience for families

In Chapter 3 I outlined some of the home circumstances in which dementing people live. I emphasized that a large minority live alone and described some types of family set-up which are frequently found. I also indicated how factors in the family structure make it more or less likely that a patient can continue to live at home, and something of how social changes are modifying these factors and are leading to greater pressures on the helping services.

In this chapter I want to concentrate more on the practical and emotional effects of having a dementia sufferer in a family, how families react and cope, and how they can be helped. Two important points need stressing.

Common reactions

In the first instance it must be realized that families vary enormously in their composition, in the personalities of the individual members, how near to the patient they live and how willing they are to help. They have differing experiences, differing family beliefs and myths and a long relationship with the affected member before her dementia began. Furthermore, they have other business on their plates as well as that of looking after the dementia sufferer.

Before examining particular family structures we will look at some of the ways in which close relatives react to dementia. Although there is a multitude of individual reactions common patterns emerge. I will describe these in terms of (1) the dying relationship (2) the changing relationship and (3) the continuing relationship. It is interesting to compare these reactions with the common reactions of the sufferers themselves (see Ch. 6). There are some similarities but many differences.

The 'duty' to care

A second point concerns the attitudes of professionals and voluntary organizations towards families. There is a tendency to assume that families *ought* to cope with dementing relatives, even if it means considerable disruption to family life, social life or work and even though the burden of caring is stressful. This attitude fits in neatly with ideas of 'community care', particularly if institutional care is seen as anonymous, depressing or degrading. But it can be a dogmatic attitude.

It is quite wrong to *assume* that a family does not care because they feel that the sufferer would be better off in a home than living with them. It may of course be true that they really do not care, could not be bothered to think of the sufferer's needs and wishes in the matter, and do not even want to think of changing their own lives to suit someone else.

But it may be that their wish not to support their relative is based on a long-standing poor relationship, which will not improve because of dementia. It may be that they really do not have the skills of patience, tolerance and humour required to cope and that they are quite right to refuse. They may genuinely feel that she would be happier and healthier in residential care. Or they may believe that it is the duty of the state to provide care for those who cannot care for themselves, and would wish the same for themselves if they became disabled. In Scandinavia and some other parts of the world, much higher percentages of the elderly live in residential or hospital care than do in Britain. In some other parts of the world the percentage is less than in Britain. There are no absolutes here, only opinions and customs.

Encouragement or pressure. We, as professionals dealing

with individual families, have no right to cajole or coerce families into coping. We can encourage them to do so if we feel they *can* cope, we can ask them to consider carefully the alternatives that are available, we can urge them to consider the wishes of the patient and most important of all we can provide moral and practical support if they *do* wish to care. But there can be no law which states that relatives ought to care.

However there *is* pressure on relatives. It may come from their own loyalty, conscience and religious beliefs. It may come from the patient's wishes or from promises given to her in the past. It may come from the expectations of other members of her family, from friends and from the community in general. Or it may come from the subtle, and sometimes not so subtle, pressures of the professions. Worst of all is the pressure that comes from lack of resources (p. 82). The common reactions of relatives seem to occur whether they are more willing or less willing to cope with caring at home.

THE DYING RELATIONSHIP

Dementia has been well described as a living death. As many aspects of personality disappear, as the ability to understand or respond to other people declines, as imagination, thinking and speech deteriorate, as the emotions become blunter or disappear altogether, there is little left for relatives to relate to. At the last stages there are only old memories, a few glimpses of the old personality, and the body of the sufferer still intact. Relatives often, therefore, describe a profound feeling of loss which is like grief (compare p. 175).

Mourning

Phases

The mourning process, following the *death* of someone close, has been described as a series of stages

Numbness. It begins with shock or numbness, a disbelief and absence of emotion which probably act to protect the relative from the strong emotions which they will later experience in a more controlled way.

Protest. Beginning to realize the fact of death brings a mixture of feelings. Usually the relative finds himself acting to avoid these feelings and, as it were, to recover the dead person. This has been called the 'protest' phase. *Pining* and *searching* behaviour, even hallucinations or feelings of the presence of the dead person can be seen as attempts, either conscious or unconscious, to put the clock back. *Denial* of the death can persist through this phase and cause delay in coming to terms with reality.

Distress. But in order to complete the process of mourning successfully the *feelings of loss* have to be coped with in a phase of *distress*. Although sadness or depression is the commonest feeling and is often very severe, other feelings also occur. *Anxieties* about being alone, or about suffering similar illness are common and may give rise to physical symptoms. *Anger* at doctors and nurses, or other relatives who are thought not to have responded may be justified or unjustified, but is often felt very strongly. So is the more surprising anger at the dead person for leaving the relative. And so is anger at the self, the relative feeling that they have somehow been at fault. These and other feelings, including envy of the dead person, gratitude for a past good relationship, joy after a bad relationship, relief after suffering and the renewal of old feelings from the past are mixed together. The result can be a bewildering, disorganized experience.

Recovery. Eventually these feelings lose their strength, or are resolved and the relative can move to the recovery phase. Now the relative must look at how his own life has been changed by the death and consider how to reorganize it so that he can continue to obtain satisfaction and happiness in a future bereft of someone very close. All the phases of the mourning process must be gone through, though not necessarily in strict sequence, if the relative is to reach a satisfactory recovery. Attempts to hurry it, to avoid the feelings, or to change nothing only delay or prolong the process.

Losses

It has become more and more clear since the phases of mourning were first defined that grief does not only follow death. It is in fact a universal process following the loss of any thing or person which has been important. The same phases and the same types of feeling are involved whether the loss be loss of self-esteem after a failed exam or a broken engagement, loss of a limb or loss of money. So the multiple losses of dementia must cause grief in close relatives.

Factors affecting mourning

A number of factors determine the *severity* of an individual's reaction to a death or other loss, and how it is coped with. The most important are the closeness and importance of the person or object lost, whether the loss was expected, the personality of the person experiencing the loss, and previous experience of loss. In assessing the reactions of relatives to dementia we will see rather similar factors operating as the person goes through the process of grief.

Mourning in dementia

Grief for dementia differs in two important ways from grief induced by the actual death of a near relative. Firstly, the person is still alive and indeed may be physically very healthy. Secondly, the process stretches over long periods of time, months or even many years.

Anticipatory mourning

Those who have studied grief reactions have described 'anticipatory grief', a working-through in the imagination of what it will be like to lose a close relative or friend. This usually occurs if the relative or friend becomes ill and death is a real possibility. But many older married people think a lot about the prospects of their partner's death and prepare for it in imagination long before it is likely to happen. Some of this anticipation of actual death must go through the minds of relatives of dementia sufferers. But as well as that there is anticipatory grief for the parts of the person that will be lost forever long before her death.

Helping anticipatory mourning. If, however, every loss of dementia is unexpected, then each time something changes a new shock occurs, and the relatives are forced to experience a long series of severe, actual grief reactions. This is one of the most compelling reasons for proper education of relatives. They need to know roughly what to expect. Then they can think out how they will feel and how they can cope practically if changes do occur. In relatives' groups, a lot of this anticipatory grief-work can be effectively carried out in a reassuring atmosphere.

Numbness and shock

The sense of *shock* when the patient's symptoms first appear, can be enormous, especially when the patient is young and the dementia completely unexpected. There seems also to be greater shock if the patient has previously been active in mind and body, outgoing in personality or organized and careful. It is almost as if relatives did not expect dementia to strike such people. Shock is greater if the dementia has been covered up by the patient herself or by another well-meaning relative and is suddenly discovered. And it is greater if the change in the patient's personality is sudden or considerable. The greatest shock of all, however, may be the discovery of the diagnosis, a situation not helped by the tendency of some doctors to avoid saying the actual word 'dementia' until a late stage.

Helping numbness. Time and a little privacy can help during the period of shock. The most useful active assistance that can be given to relatives is to show empathy, to say that it is understandable to be shocked, and to give permission, that is, to say that it is acceptable to feel this way.

Protest and denial

But shock is usually less acute in dementia because of the slow progress of the illness. A bigger problem is *denial*. Denial can be seen as an attempt to avoid the implications of loss, both the feelings and the readjustments that must be made. It is understandable except when taken to extremes. It leads relatives to deny the evidence of dementia, to explain forgetfulness or poor self-care as laziness, to cover up for the patient's lapses so well that they can ignore the evidence. It leads them to search for any diagnosis other than dementia to explain what is happening. This search is, of course, reasonable in the early stages, but later amounts to denial of the obvious. Pining and searching for the lost person are demonstrated by persisting hopes of a cure, or by claiming to see fragments of the patient's old personality long after they have disappeared. More extreme denial can cause practical and dangerous problems, for a relative who believes that there is nothing wrong with a dementing person may leave her in a needlessly risky position.

Helping denial. Denial needs sensitive handling. It is, after all, a powerful defence mechanism that people use to avoid very distressing feelings. It is unlikely to be overcome by confrontation with the facts, tempting though that may be. A gentle approach is more helpful, firstly gaining the relative's confidence, then gradually presenting the reality of the situation while preparing them for the mixed and distresssing feelings that are bound to follow when reality strikes home. Denial is often based on fear, some of which may be groundless. For example, the relative may fear that they will be left with no help, or that dementia means uncontrollable behaviour. Discussion of any such fears can ensure that denial gives way to realistic acceptance of a difficult situation.

Distress

The *feelings* which the losses of dementia arouse in close relatives depend very much on the nature of the relationship which existed beforehand, and each individual relative needs to be understood in his own right. The range of possible feelings is great. As already stressed, the prolonged nature of the illness and its gradual worsening bring the relative constant reminders of his loss.

Sadness is likely to be the predominant emotion. The isolation of having to cope alone with a partner who can no longer reciprocate support or warmth is particularly depressing. And missed opportunities or unfinished business from the past can bring nagging regrets or bitterness.

Anger can be directed at many targets — against fate or God for inflicting the illness on the patient, or inflicting the burden on the relative; against the patient, who may be accused of bringing it on herself, or of not trying hard enough; against other relatives or professionals who are seen as unhelpful; against the self in the form of guilt about real or imaginary actions or inaction, which have brought on or exacerbated the dementia. Anger is often a surprise in grief. Everyone expects to feel sad, not angry. Yet it is perfectly understandable that if our whole life has been transformed by circumstances out of our control, we should feel angry and wish to lay blame.

Anxiety is another understandable reaction to a change in circumstances when there is no certainty of what will happen. It can take various forms. The relatives may have a fear of not coping, which may or may not be realistic. Or they may become anxious about their own health. They may, half-jokingly, wonder whenever *they* have lapses of memory, if they too will 'go the same way'. Or they may become worried by the genetic risk. The extreme of this anxiety is the very real predicament of relatives of Huntington's chorea patients, who have to live with a strong possibility of developing the illness themselves (see p. 164).

Helping distress. Helping people cope with feelings of loss is largely a matter of listening. Some need to be encouraged to express their feelings because they are surprised or embarrassed by them. Support groups are of great help in giving this 'permission' to feel and to express feelings, but relatives also need prolonged individual support.

In addition, strong emotions can lead to action. Anger may lead to accusations or to violence; anxiety to attendance at the doctor for treatment of physical complaints; depression can cause relatives to feel like giving up even when they wish to go on. Workers who are giving support to carers should also be listening to these proposals for action and should spend time talking them over with the relative. They should be comparing the relative's reading of the situation with reality, and, if necessary, advising delay before action.

However, there usually *are* realistic actions to be taken, and these are the basis of the recovery phase. Listening is all very well, but it should not go on interminably. The relative should be guided towards a resolution of his feelings and on to a phase when he can deal effectively with the situation that he is in.

Recovery

For the relative of a dementia sufferer, recovery from these feelings involves coming to terms with the situation, organizing effective help and making the required decisions without being crippled by distress. It is obvious that the progressive decline of dementia, the changing situation and the multiplicity of deficits make any real resolution difficult. A new disaster comes just as the last one is being dealt with. Nevertheless, it is reasonable to attempt to get past the phase of emotional distress into a more practical phase of coping and organizing. Indeed some relatives who have expected not to be able to cope gain considerable confidence and self-esteem through resolving practical problems and proving that they *can* cope.

Helping recovery. Helping relatives through the recovery phase is largely a practical matter. It is best if possible solutions to practical problems are suggested by the relatives themselves. They feel more effective in this way and dependence on the helper can be largely avoided. For, if a relative has had a helper with a receptive ear and a sympathetic voice during his grieving, it is difficult to let go of that helper when the worst of the distress is over. He must prove that he can 'go it alone'. The helper should not be surprised, however, if some of the distress returns from time to time as recovery progresses. This is understandable, though the relative will then need encouragement to get back to practical problem-solving.

Sense of relief

This process of grieving has to be gone through to a greater or lesser extent for all the losses of dementia. Some, such as the initial diagnosis, or the realization that a relationship has disappeared for ever, or the move from home to care, will be difficult losses. Others will be minor. By the time long-term care is needed or when finally death comes, a great deal of grieving will have been done, and all that is left is a sense of relief. That in itself can pose problems, for absence of feeling after a close relative's death can make one feel embarrassed or guilty. Reassurance may be required that the sense of relief is understandable and acceptable. And, in any case, that may not be the end of the story. Even after the patient's death old feelings of guilt, sadness, anxiety or bitterness will inevitably return from time to time.

Abnormal grief

There are two important ways in which the mourning process in dementia may go wrong. Firstly, relatives may be tempted to avoid it by denial. Secondly, they may try to hurry it up by giving up coping and by wishing to reject the patient. Many of the problems which arise as families try to cope with dementing relatives and try to work with supporting services can be seen as variants of one or other of these two problems. Denial can explain how some relatives are over-optimistic about their own or the patient's ability to cope, how some will not allow services to take over part of the burden and how others disagree with or obstruct the rest of the family who are trying to seek help. Giving up too early to avoid distress can sometimes explain precipitate requests for long-stay care, impatience with attempts to plan care, or pessimism about what can be achieved. We should help relativess to go through the phases of mourning the multiple losses of dementia *at a rate that is reasonable for them.*

THE CHANGING RELATIONSHIP:
1. COPING WITH DEPENDENCE

Recovery from the realization of the many losses in intellect, self-care and personality that dementia brings must involve a change in relationship between relative and patient. The central element of this change is a move from independence to dependence on the part of the patient. Whereas she used to think independently, to look after herself, to have something to offer in conversation, to be able to fill her day with work and pastimes, she now requires someone to think for her, to look after her, and to provide activities. The change will be even more striking if, before the onset of the dementia, family members were dependent on *her*. As has been stressed so often, these changes are gradual and subtle. They tend to creep up on a family, who may respond to the change almost without knowing it.

There are two aspects to the reactions of relatives to new dependence. The first is practical, the second more to do with emotions, attitudes and roles in the family.

The practicalities of dependence

Relatives as staff

Chapter 4 indicated how family, as well as staff in home or hospital, fill the gaps in ability opened up by dementia, and Chapter 8, on decision-making, describes other types of gap which may have to be filled by relatives. Particularly where relatives live with the patient, the distinction between staff and family becomes blurred. By carrying out practical caring the family are in a sense acting as 'staff'. Or, to put it another way, the only difference between 'formal' and 'informal' carers is that the formal carers may have had a training for their job, and get paid a lot more for doing it.

Relatives are involved throughout dementia in assessing the deficits of the patient, in deciding how to fill gaps and whether to fill them, in working out who does what for the patient, and in carrying out the day-to-day work. The functions of professional or volunteer advisors are to support relatives in those tasks, to 'train' them, and to help decide which gaps are to be filled by the relatives and which by outsiders.

Training. Most of this training, support and decision-making tends to be carried out in a haphazard way, spread over several years as it must be, and divided between different advisors, sometimes with differing ideas. Some relatives will have access to a specific educational group for 'new' relatives who are having to cope with dementia for the first time. Some relatives will have a key person to whom they can refer throughout the illness. But for most, training consists of a mixture of learning by trial and error, chatting with other relatives in the same position, asking specific bits of advice from the health visitor, general practitioner or other staff, or reading a book. Several guides for carers (see Further reading, p. 317) have been published. They provide useful training for relatives, not only in the practical issues of caring, but also in learning what problems can occur, what feelings to expect in themselves, and where to go for help.

How much help? Relatives are the main providers of memory and other aids. They help with reminders of time, reminders of meals and of self-care. They help with dressing, washing, bathing and toileting. They decide things on the patient's behalf and help with paying bills. They provide stimulation and reality orientation. How much of this should they be doing?

Realistically, how much relatives do is all too often decided by the absence of services as shown in the balance of care diagram (Table 3.5), but we should be trying to get away from that as much as possible. What relatives do *should* be a considered balance between what they are able to do, what they are willing to do, and what can be offered. We should question whether an elderly or disabled spouse is physically able to bathe and dress their wife or husband, and whether a mentally handicapped daughter has the skill to deal with memory aids.

How much sacrifice? Practical caring can mean having to give something else up. Is it reasonable for a daughter to give up her work, for a husband to retire prematurely, for social life to be restricted because of the need to care for a dementing relative? We should question the willingness of relatives to give support, even when they are able and seem to be offering it. They may be offering in desperation, out of a martyred feeling of duty, out of an obligation demanded by the dementing person, or out of ignorance of available services.

How much willingness? In general, the true willingness of relatives to cope with a dementia sufferer at home depends mainly on the strength of their previous relationship. If a relative has had a good strong relationship, and feels that the patient has given them a lot over previous years together, then they will probably feel positive towards the idea of caring for her now. They will feel more sadness at the loss, but may be patient and tolerant, in a way which other relatives are not. The danger, indeed, for such relatives is that they try to take on too much and resist reasonable outside help.

If the relationship has been poor, on the other hand, there is likely to be little loyalty, so caring may be half-hearted and not carefully thought out. Such relatives are likely to want to hand over the caring to others at an early stage.

Family or outsiders? Having assessed the relatives' ability to cope and their willingness to cope, and after working out with them whether they can be trained to cope better, arranging outside help becomes a matter of filling those gaps in caring that have been reasonably left by the family.

Helping relatives fill the gaps

Intermittent help. Most of the help that patients need could be described as intermittent, and most of the help relatives need is also intermittent. This consists of help with tasks that are spread over the day such as eating, toileting, dressing, going to day care etc. The patient needs some aids, or a person to be there to supervise her in one or more of these tasks, but only at particular times of the day or night. Providing bathing assistants, a home help, or a 'tucker-in' at night helps the relatives to fill the gaps at these intermittent times but also allows them to cope better at other parts of the day.

Supervision. Even more exhausting than these forms of intermittent dependence in daily living tasks is the need for more general supervision. Some dementia sufferers cannot be left alone for any length of time. If they are, they may fiddle with electrical or gas appliances, attempt to smoke in a careless way, wander out, let intruders in, or become very distressed, going to neighbours or ringing relatives or the police for help. They need a more constant type of supervision. This is particularly stressful because the relative is not necessarily *doing* anything with the patient but must be constantly alert and may even feel like a jailer. It is most stressful when the patient needs this sort of supervision at night. The relative must stay half- awake in case she decides to go off to work, or to go 'home' in the middle of the night. So outside help with supervision can ease the burden of care enormously.

Interval dependence. A useful way to think of dependence of all sorts is called 'interval dependence' — how long a person can be left without some form of supervision. It will be seen that intermittent dependence for tasks of daily living may be long or short in interval, but it is usually predictable. So help can be organized in a regular fashion. A more persistent need for supervision may allow intervals of several hours during which the relative feels that they can go to the shops and leave the patient quietly and contentedly at home. But it may allow only a short interval, or even none at all — in other words, the patient needs constant supervision. Few relatives can tolerate this, though some choose to and some have to.

Respite from caring

To deal with both intermittent and persistent dependence the relatives need regular relief for themselves — a respite from caring. Some have the ability to give themselves a break. They develop ways of 'blowing off steam' without getting at the patient. The most effective appears to be a sense of humour. Many relatives say that they could not carry on over the long periods of caring if they did not have a good laugh at the things the patient does, and the situations they get themselves into in trying to help. Relatives' meetings are therefore often surprisingly cheerful affairs despite the horror of the situations being discussed. Others get relief by physical activity, through a hobby or through talking to someone else either about the situation or about nothing in particular. Some unfortunately *do* get relief by angry words or even physical aggression to the patient. But sooner or later most will need respite from outside.

Judging interval dependence helps in planning the help to be given. How long can the relative reasonably cope without a break? Some need an annual holiday, the patient going to another member of the family, a 'foster' carer, residential or hospital care for a few weeks. Some need a regular day to themselves when the patient goes to day care. Some need an hour or so when a neighbour, family member, or companion/sitter supervises the patient. Some need help at night, with a night sitter, a nurse or another family member providing the supervision. Some need most or even all or these. The judgement of what is reasonably offered is largely up to the relatives. They will be all too aware of what has been called the '36 hour day' of caring.

The effects of dependence

A relative may be willing and able to cope with increasing dependence. But even so changing into a 'carer' inevitably brings great changes in the relationship between relative and sufferer. People do not usually plan or choose to be carers; they have the role thrust upon them and accept it more or less willingly. And they are unlikely to foresee how it will alter their lives.

Restrictions

First, there is a restriction of social life and privacy caused by caring. Even if the relative has *chosen* to give things up this can bring hidden or open resentment, to the extent of blaming the patient for ruining a good life. There is a danger of an atmosphere of bitterness in the home, or even of violence towards the patient. On the other hand a relative may adjust to the new situation by making it their 'job' to be a carer. This enables them to cope with the more distressing aspects of caring with dispassion. The danger is that the relative becomes too business-like and emotionally detached and so neglects both his own and the patient's feelings. But in general, treating caring as a job usually has advantages for relatives. They do not resent the loss of their own independent life so much, and can usually work with outside help better (unless they have become so over-competent that they resent any outside offers of help).

Role reversal

Second, there is a reversal of roles. Very many relatives comment on how surprised they have been to find themselves becoming like a mother to their wife, a mother to their own mother, an intimate carer to a previously distant aunt. For many of the forms of assistance which dementia sufferers require are those required by a small child from its mother or father. Having to help with feeding, dressing, toileting, washing, having to find things to occupy time, having to keep a careful watch in case of danger are all familiar tasks to anyone who has had the care of young children. Carers have to discover within themselves the skill to carry out these tasks. Inevitably they find themselves tending to act in 'motherly' kinds of ways by treating the patient as if she actually was a child, using infantile forms of address, expecting childlike responses, disciplining or scolding in attempts to improve behaviour.

But there are great differences between an adult dementing patient and a small child. The patient is an adult, with a past in which she has been independent and capable to a much greater degree than now. It can be hurtful to treat someone in this position like a child. She may not be aware of her deficits, of her childishness, so treating her like an infant can give offence. She will not be able to recall the reminders, advice or punishment that a mother would give to a child, and she will not learn.

Unlike a child learning the skills of everyday life, the dementing lady is *losing* her skills, and losing them in a disorganized fashion. So although reminders and even scolding might maintain her level of functioning temporarily, it is always a losing battle, and the joy of seeing a child grow up and learn about life is missing.

The result is that treating a dementing lady like a child, while natural to some extent, and helpful to some extent, can upset her, upset a good relationship and be frustrating for the relatives. That being said, some relatives, who have lots of experience with children, or strong 'maternal' instincts, love the role of parent and many patients, particularly if they are either apathetic or euphoric, and were never very independent personalities, love the childlike dependent position.

Dangers in role reversal

Relatives should have the chance to realize how roles have changed and discuss the implications of this change. There are two types of situation where special help is needed.

Avoidance. There are those who do not like the idea of

being 'mother'. They may find, quite reasonably, that the more intimate parts of caring — bathing, help with incontinence, dressing, putting to bed — are foreign to them. This problem is often greater for men, be they husbands, sons, brothers or nephews, but is also a problem for wives and daughters who have never imagined that they would have to do these very personal things for their husband or parent. The relative may find the 'job' approach described above helpful in detaching themselves emotionally from the tasks they have to do. But they should also have the opportunity to talk over their embarrassment with other relatives or helpers.

Overmothering. At the other extreme are some relatives who tend to exaggerate the patient's degree of dependence, who infantilize her and overprotect her. The result is that she has little independent activity, no practice in the tasks of daily living, and is in danger of being out of touch with reality. Such relatives are usually avoiding some of their feelings of loss, or dealing with guilt about some neglect they blame themselves for in the past.

There is a danger for outside helpers here too. Relatives who overprotect and over-mother may resist outside help and appear much more able to cope than they actually are. Services are let off the hook. The relative may actually feel that he is the only person who can cope with the patient. He criticizes or rejects any outside helper who treats the patient as an adult. But the relative's attitude is unrealistic. Attempts should be made to encourage a more adult relationship, and to allow the patient a reasonable degree of independence. A gradual intrusion of outside support can help this type of situation. But, sadly, an overprotecting relative may be unshakeable.

2. COPING WITH NEW BEHAVIOUR

In Chapter 5 I have described some examples in which dementing people behave in ways that they never did before, through disinhibition. To relatives, the personality that they have known for many years has changed, sometimes quite beyond recognition. Of all the changes of dementia, personality change is probably the most distressing. Furthermore, it is usually totally unexpected. The *loss* of personality characteristics, even if unexpected at first, becomes more obvious and predictable as time goes on, so that the relatives prepare themselves gradually to lose touch with the patient as a person. But *new* personality traits occur in directions and at times that are unpredictable. The most unexpected changes occur in multi-infarct dementia when, suddenly after a stroke, even an apparently very minor one, there is a major change in the patient's behaviour. And the range of possible changes is wide — emotional lability, restlessness, disinhibited social behaviour of all kinds, coarsened habits, sexual demands.

Automatic reactions

After the initial shock, the most usual response of relatives to disturbed behaviour is automatic — they react directly to the emotions or behaviour of the patient. If they are already treating her a bit like a child, they may scold her. If she bursts into a temper, they argue back. If she is suddenly upset, they try to console her. They may be embarrassed by her coarsened behaviour, by her apparent rudenes or by the peculiar things that she says or does. This embarrassment may lead them to try to ignore her disturbed behaviour, or to avoid the public eye by keeping her in the house and away from visitors. Or they may simply feel disgusted and tend to reject her.

Search for meaning

Next the relatives will look for an explanation. They are unlikely to know much about disinhibition and so may blame the wrong thing. They may blame the patient herself, thinking that she is behaving inappropriately out of malice. They may guess that she is doing things she always wanted to do and think that this is her 'real' personality emerging. Or they may blame themselves, looking for something that they have done wrong which has offended her.

Reassurance

Relatives require a proper explanation of the damage done to control mechanisms by dementia. They need to be reassured that the new behaviour is nobody's fault, neither the patient's nor their own. Their feelings of embarrassment, disgust, anger, anxiety or fear need to be aired. In particular their fears about how disturbed the patient may become need to be compared with the reality of the situation. Often, permission to see the funny side of the behaviour can be a great relief, though laughing *at* the patient should of course be discouraged.

Coping

Next, the relatives should be engaged as 'joint therapists' in attempts to modify the behaviour. They can help identify the problem clearly, look for other causes, work out what makes it worse or better, try to modify the circumstances to reduce the undesirable behaviour and help increase normal behaviour. They may need specific advice about what to say to other relatives and friends and about what to do if the behaviour occurs in public, so that their lives do not have to be restricted too much. The end result should be that the relatives are less upset by the behaviour, do not take it personally, and have worked out how best to act themselves to help reduce and control it.

3. COPING WITH INTRUDERS

As the dementing person becomes gradually more dependent, the family will be likely to need more and more outside help. As long as the relatives are not trying to cope on their own too long, or trying to reject the patient too early, this help can be organized in a gradual and agreed way (if it is available!). It is important to remember that the family's relationships have previously been private, that a marriage may have been going on for 50 years without any outside help, that most people are not used to intruders in their personal business. This, of course, applies to all forms of help offered to families. But it is particularly important in dementia because the 'intruders' may have to spend a lot of time in the family house giving practical or supervisory care. And they may have to be involved in very intimate aspects of the patient's life. This can be embarrassing or disturbing to both patient and family and needs sensitive handling. As the dementia progresses this intrusion into family life will have to increase gradually.

Reactions to intrusion

The person who is coming in to help the situation may find themselves surprisingly unwelcome because the relatives are struggling with their feelings about giving up some of the care to outsiders. The family may feel guilty about not coping enough, frustrated with the situation, possessive of the relative, more competent than the outside help. Or they may be worried that this helper is at the thin edge of a wedge whose other end is institutional care. 'Intruders' need to be alert to these possible feelings, delicate about their intrusion on the family's privacy and prepared to leave some private parts of the relationship, so that they do not seem to take over everything all at once.

Sharing care

That biggest intrusion, institutional care, should be seen in the same way. There is no need for hospitals and homes to take over every aspect of the care of their residents just because they *could* do so. Relatives, particularly spouses, should be allowed some privacy together with the patient and if possible, some continuing tasks in the patient's care. Staff who treat relatives as intruders are often missing an opportunity to share care in a constructive way. Unfortunately, some relatives are put off the idea of continuing to care by a fear that they will be asked to take over completely again. Such fears should be discussed openly and proper reassurance given.

THE CONTINUING RELATIONSHIP

Despite all the changes and disruption caused by dementia, then, relatives will very often wish to continue their relationship right to the end of the sufferer's life. Continuity is easier if outside help is introduced gradually and sensitively. It is sustained by good memories from the past, by imagining what the patient would have wanted in the present situation, and by loyalty. It is also sustained by clinging to those aspects of her appearance, personality and behaviour which survive the dementia. Some couples manage to maintain an affectionate relationship or even a reasonable sexual life well into dementia. One or two old habits, turns of phrase or gestures may be all that is left of a personality, but relatives can use these as reminders of the person as she was and continue to relate. Even after the patient seems like a stranger, loyalty, memory and imagination keep relationships good, while waiting for the death of the body.

TYPES OF RELATIONSHIP AND INDIVIDUAL REACTIONS

These then are three 'dimensions' of reacting and coping: loss; a new relationship, which involves coping with dependence, new behaviour and intruders; and the continuing relationship. In different individual relatives, with different types of patient, there will be more of one type of reaction or more of another. I suggest that for each important relative, evidence of each of these types of reaction should be sought. Then the type of support and help needed can be worked out. Much of the variation between individual reactions depends on the actual family arrangement around the dementing person and some comments on a number of differing arrangements will show the sort of problems which can arise.

The married couple, one of whom is dementing

Whichever partner is the patient, this is, for obvious reasons, the strongest and most continuing relationship met with in dealing with dementia. Loyalty 'in sickness and in health' is taken seriously by many married couples, and accepting gradual estrangement or giving over care to others is particularly difficult. That is not, however, always the case. Where there has been a poor previous relationship the onset of dementia may be seen as just another problem, and it may be ignored or lead to rejection at an early stage. On the other hand, in some previously difficult relationships, where the husband who develops dementia has been aggressive, alcoholic or unfaithful, the decline in drive that is often part of dementia can actually lead to a quieter time for his wife. So it is essential to understand both the past relationship and the changes that have occurred.

The wives of dementing men often have a particularly difficult time. They may have to cope with severe restlessnes, demands for attention and irritability or aggression at a time when they may be physically frail themselves. Sexual interest may become disorganized or demanding. Attempts by the wife to calm the situation may lead to increased aggression. Furthermore, sometimes the patient fails to recognize his spouse. Life is almost impossible for a wife who is trying to remain loyal whilst she is being treated as an intruder in her own house. It is also particularly difficult if the dementia begins at a time when the couple were looking forward to a pleasant, active retirement, for disappointment and resentment can interfere with the spouse's willingness to cope

The dementing parent living with an unmarried child

The child who remains at home is often in a peculiar position. She retains some dependence on her parents but also develops an independent life of her own. If the child is left alone with a dementing parent she has to become mother to her own mother or father, and usually has to accept some loss of her own independence and restriction of her activities. Since the balance between her dependence and independence has usually been quite delicate, this change can bring bitterness and impatience into what was previously a good relationship.

The dementing parent living with a married child and family

An arrangement to have 'granny' to live with the family will usually have been made before the onset of dementia. If it is considered during dementia, there should be an opportunity for the family to discuss at length the likely difficulties of the future, how much care are they are prepared to give and what would happen if the situation broke down. All members of the family, including children, should be involved in this discussion. The daughter or son of the dementing parent should be strongly advised not to make the decision on their own. Even decisions to accept a non-demented parent into the house should only be taken when the family have discussed what would happen if dementia, or chronic physical disability occurred. And the parent must, of course, be involved in that discussion.

Dementia in a grandparent at home can bring a family together in sharing the tasks of caring. But often loyalty to the grandparent is not shared equally by husband and wife, or the grandchildren may not wish to become involved. The dementing person may make things more difficult by putting particular demands on her daughter or son, and by becoming suspicious or critical of the spouse. And the loyalty of the son or daughter is tested to the limit by the conflicting demands of parent, spouse and children.

The solitary dementing patient with a visiting relative

Relatives who do not live with the patient are in a very different position to those who do. On the one hand they may have more anxiety about what she is 'up to' when no-one is around. On the other hand they remain visitors who can get relief from caring simply by returning to their own homes. It is very important to assess the degree of commitment of such relatives, even if they are sons or daughters; to check on how much time they are actually giving to their patient and whether their judgement of the situation is accurate. It is all too easy for visiting relatives to *underestimate* the problems and risks, assuming that the patient is fine because she is always happy to see them and behaves normally when they are there. Neighbours and others may have a different story. It is also all too easy for them to *overestimate* the problems, dropping into the situation from time to time, seeing that it is not perfect and ringing all sorts of alarm bells. The latter mistake can arise from guilt in the relatives that *they* are not doing enough, from impatience or from lack of true commitment.

The large family

Large families have opportunities for real 'sharing the caring'. Some of the most effective arrangements for care are made when a number of children share the cover of a week between them, arrange meals on a rota system, have a night rota for tucking in or sitting, or take the patient to live with them in rotation. Each of these arrangements shares out the burden equally, while giving everybody relief.

More often, however, one member of the family takes on the burden of care entirely. This type of arrangement can also work well as long as the rest of the family shows their appreciation of what is being done and offer the main carer some regular relief on a daily, weekly or holiday basis. Unfortunately relationships within families are not always so neat. One 'martyr' who takes the burden of care may let the rest of the family off the hook. Or in trying to work out rotas of care some members of the family may not wish to co-operate, foreseeing possible restrictions in their own lives.

The result of having a divided family is usually an argument between those who want to support their mother at home, and those who which her to be 'put away'. The two sides may give completely different versions of the home situation. There can be considerable value in such a family having a meeting with an outside professional, who tries to remain neutral and can help to encourage a fair sharing of burden and relief.

Family situations like this can be exacerbated by the dementing mother's expectations of one particular child, usually a daughter. And if the father lives with the dementing mother he may expect far too much of the family as a whole, saying that if he copes, they should. Very often he is not coping at all.

The other problem which arises in any family caring situation is that the burden of care falls mostly or entirely on the women in the family. It is often assumed that a daughter, daughter-in-law or even a niece, and certainly a wife will cope far better and longer than a son, son-in-law, nephew or husband. Besides not being true anyway that women are always better carers, this type of attitude is unfair, and professionals should be aware of this when looking at who is available to care and what they can offer.

Staff as family

In any long-term institution it is not unusual for individual staff members to take on some of the aspects of being a relative. They too can feel the sense of loss and the difficulty of coping with caring. If they become attached to the patient they may feel that other staff 'do not understand' and become possessive. They may even feel that relatives are 'intruders'. The maintenance at the same time of both detachment and a caring involvement is one of the most difficult tasks for staff who are coping with dependent residents.

TYPES OF HELP NEEDED BY RELATIVES

Having described the differing types of reaction of relatives and the various family set-ups we can now see some important forms of help which are needed to enable families to cope.

Education and advice

Relatives need to know the diagnosis and the implications of that diagnosis. Neglecting to tell them is not a kindness, for without this information relatives have only their own fantasies to work on. Telling the facts can bring relief, and can help the family replan their own lives and look for appropriate help. They can stop merely reacting and start working.

But they need a lot of knowledge to work on. This can be given in interview or in a small group, or by learning from other families. The books listed on page 317, produced by the Health Education Council and the Alzheimer's Disease Society (ADS) are extremely helpful in introducing to relatives the stages of dementia and its associated problems, in giving advice on how to cope, and in explaining about services and legal matters. Used in the right way they are reassuring and practically helpful, even though they tell a depressing story. But families need to be warned that their relative will not necessarily present all the problems mentioned. And they should be given opportunities to discuss any worry or uncertainty that comes out of their reading.

When one particular problem becomes paramount, relatives may need special education, with a chance to learn of a variety of ways to cope, or of one specific technique which may relieve the problem. In searching for residential care, a lot of information is needed about types of home, what to look for, standards of care, money matters.

Universality

Information can bring relief to relatives in another way. Very often it can seem to a carer, especially if they are isolated with the patient, that they are alone; that no-one else can be going through the same type of experience. The information books show that this is not so. But better still, meeting other relatives who are living with the same problems can bring enormous relief. It can also be a relief to know that others are even worse off! Indeed there are some relatives who go to only one of a series of relatives' meetings because they realise at the first meeting that the problems are universal and then feel better able to cope on their own.

Support

The greatest relief of all, however, can come from knowing that one's feelings are understood and accepted as reasonable, from knowing that there is someone to talk to about how it feels to care, and from knowing that that support will usually be there when needed. The feelings may be of sadness, depression, bewilderment, anxiety, fear, amusement, frustration, anger, resentment or despair. The fears may include fears about quite severe risks to the patient. The frustration and anger may reach the point of feeling like physically hitting the patient. All these feelings may be very powerful, and all can be distressing, especially in a previously happy relationship. Indeed in some studies of families, more than half the closest relatives showed as much distress as typical patients going to psychiatric hospitals for treatment.

It takes a very patient and resilient listener to support a relative through such distress. A helper must be prepared to listen sometimes for long sessions, sometimes intermittently over years, encouraging the relative to talk about feelings that are painful, giving moral support, and understanding the causes of distress, while keeping in mind also the need for practical action.

Relief

The '36-hour' day feeling has been mentioned, but all relatives who are put in a stressful situation need some form of relief. There is an emotional relief which comes from understanding something of what is happening to the patient, from universality and from support. But relief in the sense of 'time off' is also essential. Relief care ranges from a neighbour or other family member looking in for a chat, through sitting services, home care services and through day care of various kinds, to residential care relief for short or even long periods. For some relatives it is the time to themselves that they appreciate most, for others it is the relief from tasks of caring, for others it is the chance to get right out of the situation for a while, for many it is bits of all these which help.

PROVIDING THE HELP

Self-help by relatives

Some individual relatives, particularly elderly husbands or wives of dementing patients, are very stoical by nature. They feel they have a duty to care for their spouse, they wish to do so, and pride themselves in being able to find solutions to some of the problems of dementia by themselves. This should not be decried. Presenting this type of relative with a well thought-out programme of care for the patient is not appropriate. It may indeed be considered rather insulting. Nor should we be too critical if all the relative's techniques are not exactly what we would advise, or if some are even quite eccentric. If they work and are not distressing to the patient, then why not?

What such relatives need is some moral support and encouragement. They also need to be told which type of help *would* be available should they ask for it, and given some reassurance that it is not considered a weakness to have to ask for help. A watchful eye should be kept from a discrete distance in case the relative is in fact failing to cope adequately, or is shifting the load on to neighbours, friends or other family while claiming to cope, or in case the patient is suffering in some way. This type of relative usually sees their care as a 'job' and appreciates very much being treated as a semi-professional or staff member when it comes to the time that they must hand over some of the caring.

Family organization

I have mentioned earlier (p. 210) how families can organize themselves formally to care for a dementing relative. Families are often perfectly capable of doing this without outside help. If they decide to do so, the following principles are useful. They should, if possible, hold a family meeting, so that everyone agrees together and there is a sense of a contract being made. They should consider seriously having the patient at the meeting, even if she does not fully understand, or is likely to be somewhat distressed. The fact that all the family agree to a particular arrangement or course of action can have a strong influence on whether she accepts the help offered. Decisions made behind her back are likely to be less than popular. But unreasonable distress and unreasonable pressure should be avoided. The family should ensure that *all* the important members of the family are present, and this may extend to friends and neighbours. If such an arrangement does not work they should seek outside help as referee.

Informal support

The informal and unorganized help, advice and support that family members give each other is extremely important. And the support of friends and neighbours adds to the strength of relatives in coping with difficult problems. Again, some of the advice may seem eccentric or even negative, but outsiders should always remind themselves that these supports are *normal*. We should concentrate outside support on those relatives who are isolated by having few other family members to rely on, on those who are isolated from the rest of the family by the task of caring, on those who are distressed despite good family support, and where the patient is posing particularly difficult problems.

Help for individual families

I have outlined some of the variety of reactions of families faced with the vast variety of problems of dementia. Each family has its own structure, its own rules and its own ways of coping. It is difficult to make general rules, therefore, about how and when to help families.

A helper from outside can guess that they are being of use if the relatives are getting relief by talking of how they are feeling, if problems are being discussed and solutions worked out, if preparations are being made for future changes, if effective support is being organized. If these processes are not going forwards then there should be a question about whether this sort of support is needed, or whether the right topics are being discussed. It is all too easy for a professional to listen endlessly to a tale of woe without getting on to practical decisions about how to cope. It can also be too easy to keep trying to offer a nice plan to help which suits *our* system when the relatives actually want something else, for example, long-term care.

Key worker

Since dementia is a prologned illness the best help for relatives is also prolonged. It is also rewarding and instructive for a professional helper to see a family through the long process of decline and help them cope with the varied problems that they face. General practitioners have this opportunity, though usually only intermittently. A more regular and supportive contact can be made by a health visitor, a community psychiatric nurse, or a volunteer from ADS or other organisations who acts as 'key worker'. If this supporter is welcomed in the family, is empathic and knows the local services well, so that contacts can be easily made and important information passed on, then such individual, long-term help can be invaluable. Having a key worker, the family have someone to turn to for advice when things go wrong, support when feelings run too high and help to work out what further help is needed.

It is important, though, that all other agencies involved with the patient know who that key person is, and that the key worker has some influence on these agencies. The concept of a key worker is by no means universally accepted, but is likely to become more popular in the next few years. Without someone like this, relatives have to find their way through the confusion of different organizations and professional groups unaided.

Family meetings

We will see in Chapter 9 a particular use of family meetings when major decisions have to be made on behalf of the patient. And I have already mentioned the more or less organized support which family members give to each other. In between these two there are a wide variety of situations where outside support can be given to families by setting up a family meeting. This should not be done, though, unless there is a clear agenda of issues which need to be discussed and decisions which must be made. For meetings specially set up can all too easily raise hopes of 'something being done' which are then dashed. A family meeting may be called at a *crisis* (Table 1.4) when the home situation is in danger of breaking down and new arrangements have to be made. The roused emotions and uncertainty of a crisis situation can encourage a search for new ideas and a willingness to try out new plans of care. Family meetings can also be useful if there are *disagreements* about who should be doing what in the family and resulting disorganization in the care of the patient, or if there is an excessive burden on one or two members. But they are only useful if all are willing to take part. Otherwise they can worsen family splits. A family meeting may be useful if the *relative's distress* is becoming a problem, simply to listen to the distress and look around at all alternative ways to share the burden. And when a patient enters a *new phase of care*, be it day care or residential care, a meeting with the family can help to break ice, discuss problems and aims, and ensure that family and staff are working together.

For such meetings, it is important that all the significant

family members are present. The person in charge should
have experience of working with families. Everyone present
should have a chance to have their voice heard, and shy or
distressed members may need skilful encouragement. Family
dictators, on the other hand, need equally skilful discourage-
ment. Some family members find great distress in talking
about their patient in a group, especially if she is present, and
levels of emotion can run high. The person in charge needs
to be able to recognize and acknowledge the depth of
emotion, but at the same time keep it under control. For the
purpose of the meeting should not just be to express
emotion, but to solve problems.

Relatives' groups

Relatives' groups are of two types: those for relatives of
patients attending a specific facility, say a day hospital; and
those for relatives going for help from a voluntary organization such as ADS.

Groups like these are of great importance because they can
bring together all the types of help listed above (p. 211). The
educational element can be increased by giving out information booklets or having specific speakers on topics such
as incontinence, activities, home care, residential care or the
nature of dementia. They can be used to help organize moral
support, advice and relief. They give relatives a chance to
share with each other their feelings and ideas. They can also
be a political force, where relatives get together to press for
proper services or improvements in existing services.

However, they are not a panacea. Some relatives do not like
being in a group — they feel embarrassed, shy, or antagonistic to the idea of public discussion of personal problems.
Although the group leaders can help to encourage reluctant
people to join the group and to contribute, groups are not
the answer for all. However, it is also the case that some silent
attenders can gain a great deal from the group without
contributing. For those who are unused to speaking in a
group, the use of a guest speaker to start discussion and the
encouragement of group leaders can be helpful. But there is
also need for individual help, for not everything can be done
in a group. So an informal chat after the main meeting

becomes almost as important as the group itself.

Other sorts of relatives' meeting can be more specifically helpful. It is sometimes possible to get together a group of the wives of dementing husbands, or the daughters of dementing parents. As we saw on pages 187 to 205 there are some common problems of different family set-ups. Special relatives' meetings allow for much more cohesive group feeling, since the members are sharing very similar experiences and can give stronger support to each other in working out the solutions to their very similar problems.

How much help?

Relatives differ in their demands for help of these various kinds. But demand is much less important than need. For some people almost never ask for help, yet they may be ignorant of the facts of dementia, isolated, distressed and burdened. Others seem to want endless support. We need to search for relatives in need. This implies some 'case-finding', a task mainly for health visitors who regularly visit or screen their elderly clients. It is another good reason for early referral by general practitioners of dementing people and their families to specialist psychogeriatric services. It means publicity campaigns by ADS, Health Education, Age Concern and other interested groups, telling the public what help can be available, and encouraging relatives to come for advice and support.

CONCLUSION

In general it can be said that all relatives need education at the beginning of their experience of dementia. Their need for support, specific advice and relief must be assessed in each case, and the way in which help should be given will differ from relative to relative. There are some special occasions and danger signs when extra help may be needed. These are:

1. When dementia is first diagnosed.
2. A risky home situation.
3. A sudden change in the symptoms of the patient, especially new behaviour problems arising.

4. Any change in the family, especially a sudden change, such as a death or emigration.
5. Distress in the relatives, especially anxiety, depression or anger towards the patient.
6. A move to a new level of care, say from home to day care, or from home to hospital.

8

Decision-making

It will now be clear that during the long decline of dementia a number of major decisions have to be made. These decisions are mainly about accepting outside help, so as to reduce the problems and risks that arise in the course of the illness. Since the *ability* to decide is likely to be included in the general decline there is a major difficulty for the patient in dealing with such problems or risks. This chapter discusses that difficulty.

Firstly, we will examine decision-making and how it is affected by dementia. Secondly, we will look at the types of risk which arise and how control of the patient's affairs can be handed over to others to avoid or lessen these risks. Thirdly, we will consider some ways of easing the problem of decision-making and the passing over of control, by better communication, group discussion and advocacy.

Types of decision

Two main areas of decision-making are important in relatoin to dementia. The first concerns the *financial affairs* of the patient, including the making of a will, the second concerns the *acceptance of care* by the patient in her home or in an institution, including the acceptance of medical treatment

The distinction between problems of finance and problems of care is worth making because there is a separate set of laws relating to each category, but there are many overlaps in practice. Financial decisions range from the decision about who should collect the pension to major transactions such as the selling of property and the handling of large investments. Making a will is a particular decision which requires the maker to be fully 'capable' of appreciating what she is doing. There are risks in dementia of financial neglect by the patient, of mismanagement, and of undue pressure from others. Physical risks, requiring decisions about care, include those of self-neglect, dangers in the house, maltreatment by carers, and neglect of medical care. Disagreements often arise between the patient, her family and professionals about what help if any is needed to lessen these risks. Physical risks can sometimes be matters of life and death. Decisions must be arrived at somehow.

Of course decision-making is of much more general importance. It affects every aspect of a patient's life — what she should eat, what she should wear, how to spend time and with whom, who does what in the house. Whilst our discussions will centre on the major decisions, the problems involved in making these minor decisions should always be borne in mind.

Normal decision-making

Normally an adult expects to be in charge of her own affairs — her finances, where and with whom she lives, how and when she seeks help and advice from others. In practice, of course, no-one makes decisions in a vacuum. Even if we *feel* independent, we are subject to all sorts of pressures from others and from within ourselves. How we decide on a particular issue will reflect our own experience, upbringing and attitudes. It will also be influenced by pressure from our family, friends and society at large as well as by what the law says. Furthermore, some courses of action that we would like to take may not be available to us, some forms of help not on offer.

Contracts

Nevertheless, most of us feel that we are at least *active participants* in decision-making, that we *consent* to what is done for us or in our name, and that we could say 'no' if we wanted to. We are able to enter into agreements or *contracts* with other people, though most of these contracts are implicit rather than explicit.

If a dementia sufferer needs a home help in order to survive from day to day then a decision is required. This involves an agreement that the help should come into the home, and an agreement to pay for the service. In other words a care contract and a financial contract are made. Likewise if medical treatment is required, a 'contract' is assumed between doctor and patient (though not actually signed unless an anaesthetic is required). In this 'treatment contract' the patient, having told the doctor the problem, and having been examined, is offered treatment and judges that she is prepared to accept that treatment. In going into residential care both a decision to move into care and a financial decision to pay need to be made and agreed with the home.

Even in the absence of dementia the practice and theory of decision-making and contracts can be far apart. Agreements may be reached or contracts signed under pressure. The person who makes the contract may not realize the full consequences of a particular choice. But dementia sufferers are in special difficulty in making any of these important decisions and contracts.

DECISION-MAKING IN DEMENTIA

Reduced to its simplest the process of decision-making for any individual should involve the following steps:

1. Awareness that there is a problem to be solved
2. Understanding the nature and extent of the problem
3. Consideration of possible solutions, understanding what they are and foreseeing their consequences
4. Free and informed choice of a particular solution
5. A 'contract' with whoever else is involved
6. Compliance with the implications of that contract.

In all these areas the dementing person is at a disadvantage. This disadvantage is usually said to be due to lack of *insight*, and certainly insight is important, but other changes of dementia are also involved.

Insight

We have seen earlier (p. 167) how complex a process insight is. It is the ability to appreciate that one is ill and to be aware of the degree of that illness. Loss of insight will clearly affect the first two steps in decision-making. A lady who does not think that she is ill will see no need for major changes or decisions, and if she underestimates the extent of her impairment she will wonder why people are fussing so much. We have seen how denial complicates insight and makes it difficult for us to assess it.

Understanding

As well as appreciating that she is ill, it is also important that the patient appreciates the risks that the illness has caused. To understand a risk from leaving gas taps on, or letting bogus workmen in she must *perceive* the risky situation, grasp its *meaning*, and *remember* it. All these functions are likely to decline in dementia, so many patients seem blissfully unaware of the dangers as they sit in a gas-filled house, fail to appreciate the risks of having a stranger in the house, or, if they have understood, quickly forget these risky situations and refuse to discuss the problem.

Insight and understanding

Both insight into illness and understanding of the risks are important. Some patients preserve one ability but not the other. Thus many sufferers admit to declining memory but are unable to see that this means a need for outside help. They seem unaware of the evidence of a neglected house, poor self-care, unpaid bills, and so, despite the evidence that *we* see, they claim to be managing well. It is possibly more startling if the patient seems fully aware of the mess yet still claims to be managing.

Three other deficits help to explain these situations. Firstly, there is the loss of ability to make *connections* between different areas of the brain that is required to think rationally. Secondly, because of frontal lobe damage, the ability to compare reality with a standard is damaged. The patient has a decline in *judgement* and conscience. Thirdly, the decline in *emotions* bring apathy. Even if she has insight, understands, connects these rationally and judges the situation, she may simply not *feel* much about it and so ignore the risks.

Other losses

Even if insight and understanding are good, attempting the rest of the steps in the decision-making process highlights other deficits. If she suffers *dysphasia* she will have difficulty understanding what others are saying about her problems and possible solutions, or difficulty in expressing her own conclusions. Her ability to formulate plans and solutions will be limited by deficits in *thinking* and particularly in *abstract* thinking — moving from the particular to the general becomes difficult. Indeed, she is likely to avoid working with concepts and generalizations altogether and think and talk at a *concrete* level, or in old platitudes. Thus she may be able to understand that she cannot cook safely and needs help, but be unable to generalize to the idea of having a home help, or to see the other consequences in terms of her general need for care. Indeed, she may be at the same time declaring repetitively the old platitude about 'not going into a home'. The bewildered professional who has come to assess the situation is left not knowing whether she wishes help or not. Discussion is also likely to be hampered by the problems of *attention* described in Chapter 5. She cannot focus on the decision in hand, the discussion is rambling and decisions are never reached.

Choice of a decision depends not only on insight, understanding and the ability to think, discuss and decide, but it also requires *motivation* and decisiveness. The apathy already mentioned makes patients less inclined to bother about decisions. And, of course, difficulties with *memory* can sabotage any attempt at compliance with an agreement. For even if we can hold her attention long enough to go through the groundwork and come to a rational decision, the whole process is dubious if then she quickly forgets it and disclaims all knowledge of the discussion 2 minutes later.

Disinhibition and personal reactions

Thus decision-making is imperfect because of the losses of dementia. It is also interfered with by the other changes of disinhibition and personal reaction. A decision based on totally false ideas or disturbed emotions due to disinhibition must be questioned. Many patients, aware to some extent of their dementia, become more *cautious* than they were before, because they see the danger of making silly mistakes, or being exploited. So they avoid decisions altogether or hand over too easily to others, thus actually making themselves more susceptible to outside pressure. The opposite occurs sometimes in patients who have previously prided themselves in their *independence* (p. 161). If they retain that personality trait, but lose insight they may be very strong in their wish to make decisions for themselves, but reach quite misguided conclusions. Furthermore they will resent any attempt by other people to make decisions for them, especially if this means becoming more dependent. Such patients are the most difficult of all. They live on in risky situations, insisting that they 'have always coped, so they can cope now' and refusing all offers of help, sometimes quite agressively.

Assessing decision-making

How, then, are we to judge a dementing patient's ability to decide for herself? The task of assessing whether she is aware of her illness, whether she understands the risks it has led to and whether she can manage the steps to make a valid contract is inevitably complex and imprecise. We not only need to look at the reality of the situation, what risks are involved, what help 'should' be provided. We also need to know the patient's personality and her previous attitudes to outside help; and we need to know her present deficits and the changes that have occured in her. From these we can guess what she *would* have decided if she were not ill. We also need to keep in mind both the ordinary cautiousness and rigidity of old age and changes in her attitudes which are more to do with her cirumstances than with her dementia. She may, for example, have reason to mistrust her family; she may not have anyone to confide in, or she may have particular habits acquired over years of solitary living — all these affect how she will approach big decisions.

Taking over

So difficult is it to evaluate the complex process of decision-making that it is tempting to assume that from the beginning of dementia the patient can make no decisions for herself at all. The family therefore make decisions behind her back. Care is arranged for her without discussion. Choices are not put to her. This approach is made even more tempting if the patient does not seem to object. The general lack of interest of the public in dementia and its problems means that there is little pressure to do otherwise.

Objections. There are three objections to taking over from the patient in this way. First, insight and all the other functions we have discussed are declin*ing*, not lost. At late stages they are as good as lost, and the non-communicative, emotionally bland, severely demented lady is manifestly unable to form any sort of real contract. But at all earlier stages the losses are partial and she retains some ability to grasp, reason, draw conclusions, discuss and agree or disagree. Second, if she has some remaining abilities she has the same *right* to be involved in managing her affairs as anybody else and to object to others taking over from her unnecessarily. And, of course, some patients actually do object and say so. Thirdly, there are many decisions which, in order to be *legal*, require her agreement or signature, for example, many financial transactions, the making of a will, admission to a residential home and receiving an anaesthetic.

Handing over

So, at the beginning of dementia, the patient will be making all her own decisions or will be able to agree to the decisions of others. At the end she will be totally unable to be involved.

The process of handing over decisions to others would ideally be gradual, and ideally she would be involved in the decision to hand over. Six main possible cases exist in practice:

1. The patient has good understanding of the issues and can judge and reason. She decides to hand over her affairs to someone else to allow them to make decisions for her.
2. She has good understanding etc. but refuses to hand over.
3. She has good understanding etc. but cannot communicate her views.
4. She has poor understanding etc. and agrees to hand over.
5. She has poor understanding etc. and refuses to hand over.
6. She has poor understanding etc. and cannot communicate.

The possibilities are multiplied when we consider also the changeability or indecisiveness of some patients, and the different degrees of pressure and influence of families and professionals.

Difficulties. Only case 1 represents a proper contract. In case 2 we ought to take account of the patient's wishes, though this is not always done. In cases 3 and 6, we have no idea what her wishes are. Too often her lack of communication is taken to mean agreement. We make decisions that are guided by guesswork, her previous wishes or what suits others. Compulsory powers, which should at least be considered, rarely are. In case 4, agreement is usually, quite wrongly, taken at face value. So it is only in case 5 (and occasionally case 2) that the possibility of a compulsory take-over is even considered, and often it is dismissed. The result, as we shall see, is that very little formal discussion of decision-making occurs and remarkably few dementing people who are unable to make their own decisions have proper legal protection.

RISKS

Discussions about whether the patient can decide for herself or whether others must decide for her usually concern situations of risk. Before discussing the practical aspects of decision-making, we will therefore examine these risks.

There is a wide variety of risky situations that dementing people can get into. In each situation, the decision that must be made is whether (i) to leave her in charge and accept the risk, (ii) to persuade her to accept help to lessen the risk, or (iii) to take control out of her hands by compulsory means. What is actually done will depend on the degree of risk involved, which of the 6 categories the patient is in, the feelings of everybody else involved in the situation and the powers available. As emphasized in Chapter 3, availability of help may actually be a bigger factor than any of these in deciding what is done. If a lady needs a hospital bed, and does not want it, but it is not available anyway, then she will stay at home whether we like it or not. Despite this reality we should not be prevented from a proper assessment of the situation.

FINANCIAL RISKS

The dementing person is likely to *neglect* to collect her pension, or neglect to pay bills for gas, electricity, rent, rates, etc. She may miscalculate how much money she has in the house. She may make mistakes in shops. Simple memory impairment and loss of the ability to calculate (dyscalculia) are not the only problems however. If memory impairment is linked with a little *disinhibition* the patient may withdraw money repeatedly from the bank, pay the same bills again and again, or hand out large sums of money to others. Loss of concern and carefulness, together with poor understanding of the value of money and possessions, leave the patient open to *exploitation* by bogus workmen who charge excessively, or by bogus salesmen who offer tiny sums for valuable furniture or clothes. Exploitation also occurs when friends or relatives get her to sign cheques for them, give them money, change her will in their favour or sell her house, when she has little idea of what she is doing. *Hoarding* of large sums of money, and *miserliness* over bills is common. These habits probably arise early in dementia when the patient realizes that something is wrong and wants to protect herself against making mistakes or being exploited (compare p. 183). Memory impairment and *paranoid thinking* can lead to mistaken ideas that the home help, the family or others are stealing from her. Telling the difference between real and imaginary stealing is often very difficult indeed, and such situations need to be handled very sensitively.

The risks of neglect, mismanagement and exploitation are obvious. In some ways richer people are more at risk, for they have more complicated financial affairs and are more tempting targets for exploitation. But people with little money run exactly the same types of risks and deserve similar sorts of protection.

Reducing financial risks

How can the patient or others take decisions which will reduce these risks and ensure the protection and proper management of her financial affairs and property?

Informal arrangements

A person who cannot get to the post office can sign over the right to collect her pension to a relative or friend. She should be able to understand that this is happening. If someone is unable to pay her bills then a bank manager may be prepared to arrange informally for their payments if a relative sends them in. Standing orders or direct debit arrangements allow regular payments to continue. But informal arrangements like this are dangerous. Unscrupulous relatives or friends can apply undue pressure or manipulate the arrangement for their own ends.

Institutional arrangements

The staff of a residential home can manage the day-to-day financial affairs of residents, and have a duty to ensure that they have a certain amount of 'pocket-money' each week. In hospital, pension books can be taken over and the patient's finances can be run by the hospital management. Continuity of family relationships (p. 206) can often be maintained better, however, if relatives are allowed to go on managing the finances of the patient after admission to care, though they may need reminding of the regular clothing and comfort needs of a long-stay resident.

Most of these arrangements assume the consent of the patient. It is assumed that she cannot manage her own affairs but can *instruct* others in their management (category 1 on p. 227). Theoretically she has instructed the family or the institution to manage her affairs for her.

Power of attorney

This same theory applies to power of attorney, invented originally to cover temporary physical illness, where the patient was unable to go about her financial business and needed someone to stand in for her. She could make the other person her 'attorney' with full powers over her financial affairs by signing a legal document to this effect. When well again she would take back control.

Validity. In order to sign a valid contract the patient obviously has to be able to understand what she is doing, what her 'affairs' consist of and who she is granting them to; and she must continue to understand in order to be able to revoke it. As a general rule, therefore, people who are dementing would be unable to sign power of attorney. But many have done so, and the vast majority of these arrangements have worked well and have not been challenged. But they are open to challenge as the patient becomes more and more impaired mentally.

Enduring powers. This problem has now been overcome to a considerable extent by the development of 'enduring' power of attorney, available in England and Wales. A patient, as long as she is competent when she signs, can grant power of attorney which lasts throughout her illness, even after she can no longer understand her affairs.

Compulsory powers

A patient who can neither manage her affairs nor instruct someone else to manage them is in danger of mismanaging her money herself and of exploitation by others. She needs protection. And if she is unwilling or unable to give her affairs over to someone else voluntarily this must be done compulsorily.

Court of Protection and Curator bonis. In England and Wales this is done by an application with medical evidence to the Court of Protection, a branch of the High Court. Normally the Court passes the power to a relative, accountant or lawyer who acts as 'Receiver' on behalf of the court. Or the Court may manage the affairs themselves. 'Visitors' from the Court visit Receivers on a regular basis to check that the patient's affairs are being managed correctly. In Scotland the Court of Session, following an application and the medical evidence of two doctors, appoints a 'Curator bonis' who has to report annually to the Accountant of Court on their management of the patient's affairs.

In both cases the main aims are the protection of the patient's estate intact, as well as providing for her needs. So Receivers and Curators are expected not to invest patient's money in risky ventures, or make major changes in its use. For example, selling her house because she no longer needs it is a decision which requires special consideration.

Limitations. There are two main problems with these procedures. Firstly they are expensive. If the patient has capital of less than several thousand pounds the costs of protection will eat gradually into her estate, defeating the purpose. Legal aid may be available to cover some but not necessarily all of the expenses. It is unfair if the less well off are thus excluded from proper financial protection.

The other problem is that the powers apply purely to financial decisions. It is therefore wrong if they are used to force a patient to sell her house against her will in order to force her to enter residential care. Despite these drawbacks protection of this sort is most important for the dementing and, if anything, could be more widely used.

Making and changing wills

Since dementia leads to the death of the sufferer, it is important that she has made her will. If this has happened before the onset of the illness and there are no changes in her circumstances *during* the illness, there is no problem.

Problems arise in two ways. Firstly, if no will exists the patient may herself decide to make a will or she may wish to change a previous will. Secondly, the solicitor, family or friends may suggest the need for a will, or the need to change her existing will. Is she able to make the judgements required to make or change her will? Is she open to pressure and suggestion because of her dementia? These questions are sometimes only asked after the patient's death. Then the will can be contested on the grounds that she did not have 'testamentary capacity', that is, she made or altered a will while incapable of doing so. To make a will, one must know roughly the size and nature of the estate and who are the possible beneficiaries. One must also be able to make judgements for oneself, not be abnormally suggestible, and one must be free from undue pressure. Testamentary capacity is likely to be lost relatively early in dementia.

As a general rule it is better to dissuade dementing people from making or changing wills and to question any attempt to do so. To some extent it is a solicitor's task to know whether their clients are capable enough, but where there is any doubt an examination of the patient's mental state by a psychiatrist and an opinion on their capacity should be recorded. Later disputes can thus be lessened.

The worst problems arise when an old lady has already got into the habit of will-changing or has been open to a number of pressures from a warring family. Solicitors and professional carers must protect anyone whose judgement is impaired from undue pressure from others and from their own dithering.

PHYSICAL RISKS

The central impairments of dementia and the decline in personal habits mean that many patients are at risk of self-neglect and forgetfulness. Malnutrition, unnoticed constipation, poor mobility, untreated incontinence, undeclared physical illness are all common results of self-neglect. Forgetfulness around the house brings particular risks — leaving gas on unlit, forgetting to turn electric appliances off, leaving water running, leaving the door open. Forgetfulness, together with loss of self-concern, and loss of the ability or motivation to react or complain put the patient at risk from muggers, intruders in the house, family violence and occasionally sexual abuse. Family violence may be provoked by the patient's changed behaviour and, as with violence to children, or indeed all domestic violence, is often concealed. As well as mugging, other risks can occur outside the house. Wandering can put patients at risk, especially, of course, in winter or at night. Road sense may be lost. Or a dementing person may be driving their car with considerable impairments of reaction time, spatial sense, memory or judgement.

Such risks are not confined to the patient living at home. An institution where standards or care or staff morale are low may put its residents at risk of neglect or even of physical abuse.

Reducing physical risk

Consent by the patient

Many patients accept the need for extra care and attention as their dementia progresses or do not object to others taking the decisions for them. They are in categories 1,3,4 or 6 of the list on page 227. Such patients are likely (if they are able) to agree verbally or to sign contracts which accept care or supervision in the home, day care, institutional care or medical treatment. There are dangers of coercion and of false contracts being made, but if the patient goes along with what is decided without protest there is little likelihood of any challenge. The result is that much care and treatment is given 'in good faith'.

It is possible to defend much that is done in this way even when true consent has not been given by the patient. Relatives who arrange for the gas mains to be turned off when the home help is not present, relatives who lock the door at night to prevent wandering, relatives who bring patients to day care by telling white lies, and hospital wards or homes which have locked doors or complicated devices to prevent wanderers wandering are all in somewhat the same position legally. They may be restricting the rights of a patient without her consent. But they can claim that they do these things in her best interest. And few will complain.

Consent by others

Consent given by a relative or the person in charge of the patient's care may be accepted. It is sometimes used, for example, when a patient needs a surgical operation which requires consent for an anaesthetic. It can be used when alterations have to be made to a house to improve safety. Perhaps wrongly, many admissions to hospital, be it a general, geriatric or psychogeriatric hospital, are of this general kind, where the decision is not really made by the patient but by doctors and relatives acting informally on her behalf. But we should not be complacent about doing things on 'behalf' of other people. We may be well-meaning, but we may not always be acting in the patient's true best interest. The 'rightness' of each situation must be considered individually.

The patient who refuses help or treatment

If risks are present and the patient is in categories 2 or 5, that is, she is refusing help, then compulsory powers may be considered. But these should really only apply in category 5 for in category 2 the patient, who seems to understand the situation, has decided to refuse offers of help and this may be an entirely rational decision. This particularly applies to medical decisions, when a patient may see that she has not long to live, knows that her mental powers are failing and wishes to die. She may then refuse treatment or care. Other possible reasons for a negative response should always be sought. Is the patient suffering from depression? Is her pessimism due to the discomfort of her physical illness? And how the decision will affect others should also be considered. If her decision means staying at home, does it put others at risk? Do relatives agree? Further, how major the treatment would be may be important. It may be reasonable to avoid very complex treatments which have some risk attached, while pressure may be put on the patient to accept simple treatments which would improve her comfort or quality of life considerably.

The wish to die. There are some patients who 'turn their face to the wall', (see p. 178) but they deserve a full assessment of their situation before the decision is reached that this wish to die is rational. The position of a person who, *before* her dementia began, expressed a wish not to be treated if she became demented is different. Some assessment needs to be made of whether we would expect her still to feel the same way now that she is suffering from dementia. If it is thought that she would, then her wishes must be taken into consideration as an important factor (though by no means the only one) in deciding to treat or not. Positive euthanasia is not a possible option. Those who express the view that dementia sufferers should be 'put down' are usually expressing their own impatience with 'caring' or a horror of dependence, and are misunderstanding the subjective experience of dementia for the sufferer.

But the decision not to treat is often taken by doctors and nurses.For a patient who is severely demented and unable to express a wish (category 6) it can be reasonable and humane to consider that a chest infection or the like is evidence of the body's failing ability to survive. It may then be decided, always after consulting the relatives, that treatment would not enhance the quality of her life and would needlessly prolong suffering in a fatal illness. These should be no general rule about this in a ward or a home. A decision should be made, after consultation, about each patient as an individual.

Compulsory medical treatment

If the patient is at home and neglecting herself badly, the compulsory power in Section 47 of the National Assistance Act may apply. This allows a person who is infirm (which could mean either physically or mentally), living in squalor and refusing necessary treatment or care to be removed to a suitable place for a limited period. This power could occasionally apply to dementia but is very rarely used. Thus the only powers that exist to treat a dementia sufferer medically when she has refused or is unable to give consent are the common law right to save life and protect people from injury or danger, the informal consent given by relatives and this rarely used compulsory power. All other treatment given without proper consent is given 'in good faith'.

Compulsory psychiatric treatment

There are more clear laws about psychiatric treatment. If a patient suffers from a 'mental illness' (which can include dementia) *and* there is risk to her health or safety, or to the health and safety of others due to that illness, *and* if she requires or would benefit from treatment in hospital (which can include psychiatric nursing care) *and* she refuses this treatment, then certain compulsory powers can be used. These are laid down in Sections 2, 3, 4 and 5 of the Mental Health Act (Sections 18,26 and 24 in Scotland) which cover admission for observation or assessment and admission for short-term and longer term treatment. Planned admissions follow the application to the courts by a relative or a specialist social worker (called an approved social worker in England and Wales and a mental health officer in Scotland) supported by two medical recommendations. The emergency or short-term orders require fewer formalities but must be reviewed very quickly. If necessary, an application is then made for a longer term order.

Safeguards. The powers in the Mental Health Act are great. But they are surrounded by a complicated system of reviews and appeals and by the general supervision of an independent body called the Mental Health Act Commission (Mental Welfare Commission in Scotland). These powers, therefore, at the same time take away the independent rights of the patient, and protect her right to proper care and attention.

Limited use. In practice, although these powers are often considered for dementing patients, they are rarely used. Although many dementia sufferers are at risk because of their dementia and refuse help, often the care they need is not psychiatric treatment or nursing, it is a more general form of care which does not quite seem to justify the very wide and formal powers of the Mental Health Act. This attitude may be mistaken, for the alternative is that decisions are often made behind the patient's back, subterfuges used to get her into care, or else that the risky situation at home is allowed to continue. What is more, many patients, once they are in the door of hospital settle remarkably well despite earlier protests. Whilst this can be used as an argument for not bothering to use compulsory powers, it can also used as an argument for their brief use to get the patient out of the risky situation into a safer hospital situation.

Guardianship

The 'admission' sections of the Mental Health Act cannot be used to ensure treatment of medical conditions unless they are secondary to the dementia. Nor can they be used to ensure proper supervisory care at home, or to admit someone into a residential home or an ordinary nursing home. However in Sections 7 and 8 (Section 37 in Scotland) the power of Guardianship is described. This can be of use in organizing proper general care for the patient. The procedure is the same as for Section 3 (Section 18) but in this case the court, instead of arranging admission, arranges for the appointment of a 'guardian'. This can be anybody who is deemed suitable to act in this way, but is often a social worker.

Powers of the guardian. The guardian has powers to insist that the patient allows entry to professionals who are giving or supervising her care and treatment. The guardian also has the power to insist that she lives in a particular place. This power has been used to arrange admission into residential homes. It should, however, only be used in this way after all other avenues have been considered and in practice it is much more often thought of than actually applied. Its effectiveness depends on co-operation between the relatives, the guardian and the services which are trying to provide care for the patient.

THE PRACTICE OF DECISION-MAKING

We have seen a number of circumstances where decisions must be taken away from a dementing person. At the other extreme we have seen that some patients retain, for a time, their ability to make reasoned and reasonable decisions. Between these two extremes there are considerable difficulties.

For financial decisions, power of attorney often bridges the gap, and enduring power of attorney can be continued beyond the stage of incompetence in decision- making. But, of course, not everybody has an attorney. For other decisions either the patient in theoretically is charge, or she is incapable, in which case the decision ought to be taken away from her by legal means. The gap is in practice filled by the goodwill and good judgement of those around the patient. They make up for the patient's loss of reason just as memory aids fill the gaps in her memory.

This may look good on paper, but there are many occasions when it is unsatisfactory. What if it means that unscrupulous relatives are making decisions against the patient's interest behind her back? What if the patient sees things differently from relatives or staff and wishes to argue? What if there are no relatives of goodwill around? What if the relatives disagree with each other or if professionals and relatives disagree? Who is to judge what is right? Who is to make sure that the patient's interests are protected? Who is to ensure that decisions that need to be made *are* made? It should surely be unnecessary to go to the extent of taking legal powers over the majority of day-to-day decisions. It should be possible to trust husbands or wives, children, professionals to act in the patient's best interest in most things. What follows applies mainly to those cases and points of decision where there is doubt or disagreement.

Communication

Making decisions for the patient

A relative who judges on his own how much a patient can decide, and then either makes decisions for her, or leaves her to look after her own decisions can be vulnerable on either count. In the first instance he may be accused of usurping the rights of the patient. In the second, he may be accused of putting her at risk by neglect. The same vulnerability applies to staff members who make judgements in isolation about the patient's ability to decide things.

Individuals 'get away' with these judgements for a variety of reasons. Firstly, and most important, dementing patients do not usually complain about someone else deciding for them because they are losing the ability to perceive their situation and the ability to state clear opinions, or because they forget what has happened. Secondly, the goodwill of relatives or staff is very often assumed. Thirdly, and unfortunately, other relatives or professionals may be careless about the rights of the dementing, and feel that it is not worth questioning decisions that are made.

Usually, therefore, difficulties only arise when there is a major disagreement between some of the parties concerned — the patient, relatives, staff. In reality we should *always* be aware of the problems that can arise if others make decisions on behalf of the patient, even if the person involved is a husband who appears to have his wife's best interest at heart, or a highly respected staff member, or even if the patient herself appears not to be complaining. The decisions we are talking about may have major implications for the health, welfare, or safety of a human being who may be neglected, put at risk or exploited by those nearest to her.

Talking together

The simplest way to get around this problem is to communicate, both with the patient and with other people concerned. The basic question is 'Do you agree with my judgement?' If all the people concerned are in agreement about something, then they can work together better and accusations of self-interest are much less likely. So, when we see that a decision has to be made, or is being made, either by the patient or by someone else on her behalf the best thing to do is to discuss it. But what if there is disagreement? Simply asking 'why are we disagreeing?' may resolve the issue, but if there are more fundamental or persistent disagreements, a formal meeting of those involved, a case conference, is justified.

Case conference

A case conference is advisable in three circumstances:

1. Where there are disagreements about the patient's care, or about her ability to decide for herself.
2. Where there is uncertainty or dispute about who should be responsible for different aspects of her care.

3. Where a major decision has to be made about the patient's future, because of a change of circumstances, or increased risk, and she has reduced ability to decide for herself.

Who attends?

A clear decision should be made beforehand about whether the patient herself should attend all or part of the meeting. Whatever happens, she should always be informed that it is happening and of any decisions made.

A case conference will be limited in its value if some important people are missing. It can be worth expending some effort to find all the people who regularly visit the patient or are closely involved with her, not only including the nearest relatives, home help, health visitor, GP, social worker and hospital staff, but remembering also close friends, neighbours, more distant but important relatives, clergy and church visitors, voluntary workers and solicitors, if any of these are closely involved in her day-to-day life. Small decisions may justify only a small meeting, or contact by phone. But important decisions deserve the formal collaboration of all concerned.

That being said, the most important consideration about such a meeting, which will take a number of people from their work to spend a considerable time in discussion, is whether there is adequate reason for having it at all. Case conferences get a bad name if they are used for trivial decisions or are indecisive. Whoever calls such a conference should formulate clearly what has to be decided, and why it needs the time of so many people. In these ways meetings can be shortened and made more effective.

The agenda

This should consist of:

1. Formulation of the problems, each participant getting a chance to present his/her views.
2. Clear description of the options for action (or inaction) and their likely consequences.

3. Decision-making
4. Summary by the chairman.

The chairman's role

It is the chairman's task to ensure that these four stages are gone through fully, kept separate from each other and limited in time. He has a special task in helping relatives and the patient, if she is involved, for they will not be used to speaking in a group, and may feel embarrassed. Relatives are also likely to be more emotionally involved in the problems being discussed and need protection from feeling that they are being pressurized when vulnerable or exposed to ridicule. They need to feel that their voice is being heard amid those of more sophisticated professionals. On the other hand the outcome should balance the views of *all* parties concerned and no- one should be allowed to 'bulldoze' others into a particular course of action by emotional pressure. Finally, the chairman should provide a clear account of the proceedings, sending copies to all concerned including the relatives, and even the patient, or at least communicating the decisions to her. It will be seen that such conferences will only work if the co-ordinator can be relatively unbiased and clear thinking. Flexibility is also required, for in practice it may be necessary to move more freely between the different stages of the process as participants recall more of their experience or feelings, or try to move on to decision-making too early.

The outcome

A number of types of decision can emerge from such conferences:

(i) Often no change is made. Nevertheless, there can be great benefit if the relatives feel that their concerns have been understood or shared by professionals, and if there is a feeling of solidarity in allowing a somewhat risky situation to continue.

(ii) Lines of responsibility may be clarified, communications improved, and limits set on how long the present arrangements should continue, or in what circumstances further changes need to be made. One way of ensuring a good outcome in this respect is the appointment of a 'key worker' (see also p. 215). This can be anyone who is in regular contact with the patient and who takes the responsibility of monitoring the situation — checking that services are provided and that supervisory care is maintained, continually assessing the risks of allowing the present situation to continue, looking for any change in that situation, if necessary contacting other people to review it and eventually recalling a case conference to renegotiate the decisions made.

(iii) Changes in the level of support may be organized. This may involve relatives offering more time or it may mean that they are able to withdraw more. It may mean the start or increase of home help, sitting, nursing or medical supervision, or day attendance. It may mean the supply of aids in the home or of incontinence services. Or it may mean major decisions about a move from home to residential care or hospital, or from institutional care to home.

If there is uncompromising disagreement between the patient and everybody else, with regard to financial matters or major decisions about care, then the conference may have to consider compulsory measures. Most usually the idea of compulsion can be considered and rejected. Relatives or others who feel that 'something must be done' see the consequences and limitations of compulsion and can consider alternatives. But when compulsion is necessary, then a conference decision gives confidence to those involved in carrying it into action and allows co-ordinated preparation if, say, a place in residential care or hospital is to be sought

The value of conferences

Each of these decisions can of course be made without recourse to a case conference, and only where they would otherwise be avoided or could be challenged is a conference really justified.

Much of the purpose of the conference is to smooth out disagreements. The worries of those who think that not enough is being done may be lessened if they see that the other participants are agreed on a particular course of action and most especially if arrangements are made to review the decisions of the conference at a later date, or to set limits on acceptable risks. The worries of those (including the patient) who may think that decisions are being made against her interest can be lessened by the open agreement of the participants that the action taken is necessary, and that there will be safeguards and review. Often relatives have been unhappy about explaining their fears to the patient. Although it can be very upsetting, the clear statement of concern by an important person in the patient's world can have great influence.

But a case conference should not be used to pressurize a patient into a decision for the convenience of others. If disagreements persist, compromise and later review may be only course open.

HEARING THE PATIENT'S VOICE

In all that has been said so far, the greatest danger is that the patient's voice will not be heard, or will be overridden in argument. In many cases the patient is not directly consulted at all. Who then is to speak up for her?

The patient herself

In early dementia, especially where personality is preserved, it may be perfectly possible for the sufferer to state clearly what she wants to do. There is a danger that no-one listens, particularly if she has difficulties in communication, and that can be very frustrating for her. Both relatives and staff need constant reminders that a dementia sufferer can express choice, can be involved in decisions, and generally can be an active participant in her own life. They need reminders that participation can bring enormous satisfaction to someone who fears that her competence is failing. They need to be reminded that rational disagreement is perfectly possible.

Guessing the patient's view. At later stages, and if there are severe communication difficulties, it becomes difficult to perceive what view the patient is expressing. Often a look at her *past* decisions and preferences will show quite clearly what she would wish to happen now, a further example of how essential it is to know about her past life. On the other hand such extrapolation from past to present can be dangerous. We have seen the awful position of a daughter who has been forced to promise never to 'put me in a home' (p. 210). We have also seen the difficulties posed by patients who in the past have asked to be allowed to die or even to be 'put to sleep' if they develop dementia (p. 235). We should always remember that we cannot anticipate how we will feel in the future. In particular we can have little idea what the experience of dementia will be like. And the needs and wishes of those around us are also important. So the present situation is the most important consideration, involving a balance between the needs and wishes of the patient, the needs and wishes of those around her and the judgement of professional services involved.

In severe dementia, it is almost impossible to guess at the patient's present wishes. It becomes more and more important that someone speaks wisely on her behalf.

Relatives

Relatives are in a special position with regard to a dementing person. They know what she was like before the illness and therefore are likely to understand the changes in her abilities and personality more than professionals can, and often more than the sufferer herself. They also have greater or lesser degrees of loyalty to their ill relative. They may, therefore, feel with considerable justification that they can understand what the patient's interests require and can act on her behalf — as her advocates.

Conflicting interests. Their own interests, the disturbance to their lives and the stress of caring can, however, lead to requirements which conflict with the needs of the patient. It is possible for relatives to imagine that they are acting on the patient's behalf when in fact they are pursuing their own needs. We should not exaggerate the importance of this, but it needs to be noted for it can put relatives in a difficult position

Conflicting relatives. Sometimes there is conflict between two sets of relatives, each claiming to act in the best interest of the patient. This type of conflict is likely to be greater when the stress on the relatives, or one particular member of the family is very great, where some of the family have high expectations of health or social services, or where the patient cannot express her needs clearly. In these cases professionals need to pay special attention to the separate needs of the patient herself, and emphasize to the relatives that the correct course of action is likely to be a compromise.

Relatives as advocates. It would be wrong, however, to dismiss relatives as advocates. In reality they act in this way constantly. It is they who usually bring the patient to medical attention, who ask for services, who complain when things go wrong, who assess changes in the situation, who demand action when the patient is at risk. The existence of the Alzheimer's Disease Society, many initiatives for day, sitting or other care services and much general political pressure depend entirely on the advocacy of relatives who care about obtaining proper respect and care for dementia sufferers. Only when this advocacy is absent because there are no available relatives, or when relatives appear to have negative views of the patient or do not understand her condition, or when relatives disagree need outside advocacy be considered.

Professionals

Most people who work with the elderly are committed to this work. Their interest and expertise show where help is needed, where improvements could be made, where abuses are occurring. On behalf of dementia sufferers they are advocates within their professions and organizations. Most of the pressure to improve resources for dementia in the health and social services and the drive to improve standards of care comes from those who work from day to day with dementia sufferers. This general advocacy will gradually lead to a greater concern for the rights and needs of individual patients, though at present the fact that the *amount* of resources rarely meets the size of the problem is the more pressing issue.

Professionals as advocates. On the individual level professionals and voluntary workers are often advocates for sufferers. They are advocates when they point out to relatives that the mildly demented person can still express her wishes and be involved in decisions; when they encourage a 'person-alized' approach to care, with choice, privacy and as normal an environment as possible; when they highlight the exist-ence of problems and stimulate the necessary action; when, on the other hand, they resist rushing prematurely into 'doing something' in a crisis without due consideration. In all these cases a professional or volunteer can be seen to empha-size the importance of the sufferer's rights when she cannot do this herself and when there are other, opposing influences — the wishes of relatives, the tendency in institutions to have convenient but depersonalizing routine and the pessimism and lack of imagination that is 'ageism'.

Conflicting interests. The compulsory powers discussed above have similar aims — in financial matters ensuring the protection of the person's money, in Mental Health Act matters ensuring proper care and treatment on her behalf. In these formal cases there are safeguards against abuse. But as with relatives, the professional or volunteer acting as *informal* advocate may have conflicting interests or attitudes, or be in conflict with their colleagues and others. Institutionalizing attitudes, laziness, impatience or lack of understanding can all interfere with impartial decisions about 'what a patient would like', 'what her best interests are', 'what is good for her.'

Conflicting theories. Furthermore theoretical stances can lead to conflict. An attitude which stresses the rights of the individual, though it is much needed on behalf of dementia sufferers, can tempt one into playing down the wishes of rela-tives or the stresses on them. The same can be true of those who have a theoretical objection to institutional care. Those who campaign for burdened relatives are in danger of playing down the rights of the sufferer. Those whose loyalty is to their own institution may pay too little attention to the rights of both patients and relatives. It is no wonder that steering an unbiased course and still being decisive is difficult.

Advocates

Because of these difficulties many have been considering whether some form of outside advocacy system might be useful. We could hope that between relatives and professionals the true interests of the patients would be preserved, but sadly this is not always true. There are circumstances where there are particular dangers. First there is the dementing lady living alone, in an increasingly risky situation, with worried neighbours and a not too close family. Second, there is the lady with few or no relatives, especially if she is in a large institution or in a private sector residential or nursing home. Third, there are cases where the patient's voice may not be 'heard', for example the lady living with a family who may be neglecting or abusing her. In these situations the dementing patient is open to neglect, poor standards of care, physical abuse or exploitation and she is likely to be unable to complain. If she *is* able to complain, her complaints may be ignored.

The following possibilities have been considered:

(i) A variant of the Ombudsman who would be available to look into complaints of neglect or maltreatment. Someone would still, however, have to be prepared to initiate the complaint on the patient's behalf.

(ii) An extension of the type of provision suggested in the Disabled Persons Bill to allow the appointment of 'representatives' to act on behalf of dementing patients who are unable to appoint someone themselves. Such a representative would have to be in a position to assess the situation properly and to ensure that necessary help was provided. This idea begs the questions of who would appoint such representatives and how they would have any power.

(iii) An extension of guardianship to allow guardians to act in more varied ways on the patient's behalf. This would necessitate a much more widespread use of this compulsory power. This might be seen by some as lessening the patient's right to decide instead of protecting her.

(iv) A 'panel' system, equivalent to the Scottish Children's Panel. Anyone concerned about neglect, exploitation, abuse or other risks to a dementing person could approach a local panel, which would have power to investigate the situation and could put pressure on those involved to improve the situation. The panel might even have compulsory powers. This would be a completely new venture and would require considerable organization and expense. The 'dementia team' (p. 311) could act informally in this way (though of course with little actual power except that of its members as individual professionals).

CONCLUSION

None of these suggestions is a reality. But unless some change in this type of direction occurs, many dementing people will remain vulnerable to neglect, abuse, and exploitation. We must continue in most cases only to trust to the goodwill of relatives and the wisdom of professionals. Thankfully that goodwill and that wisdom do exist in many cases and in many places. When they are absent or when the patient is not heard, advocacy and proper legal protection are needed.

9

Assessment and management

We have discussed a wide variety of problems that relate to dementia; wide because the brain is a very complicated organ; and wide because people and families are of many different types, reacting in different ways to a dreadful illness. How are we to collect together all the facts about a particular patient and her situation in a way that is both concise and comprehensive? This the job of assessment.

Assessment

The word 'assessment' has developed something of an aura around it. To some it has become the magic answer to difficult situations. But, to be worthwhile, every assessment should have a reason behind it — it should be *assessment for a purpose*. Some action should follow logically from it, and that action should benefit the patient. It is, for example, relatively useless to diagnose which type of dementia a patient has if making the diagnosis has no useful consequences for her. We should question the use of expensive diagnostic tests if they lead to diagnosis but no treatment. In a similar way, knowing the severity of dementia may not be very important in deciding placement or management of the patient (p. 76). So we should always question the time and energy that is

Stages	Methods						
	History from patient	History from relatives	Mental state	Physical state	Rating scales	Screening and special tests	ADL assessment
Baseline (before dementia began)	+	+					
Diagnosis of dementia	+	+	+	+	+	+	
Type of dementia	+	+	+			+	
Severity	+	+	+		+		+
Problems	+	+	+		+		+
Problems not due to dementia	+	+	+			+	

Fig. 9.1 Diagnosis and assessment of dementia — an outline of the stages of diagnosis and the methods of assessment. A '+' shows which methods contribute to each stage of assessment

spent on assessment rather than on doing things with the patient. In this chapter we will look at the stages of assessment and how information can be obtained for each of these stages (Fig. 9.1). This will lead on logically to a summary of management techniques (Table 9.7).

THE STAGES OF ASSESSMENT

Background information

The patient's life before the illness

This is the *baseline* from which all other information is judged. We cannot say that someone is changing unless we know what they were like before. We cannot expect to re-habilitate a patient to a better level of function than she started with — whether in breadth of interests, activities, level of self-care or intellectual ability. (I have mentioned elsewhere (p. 208) the rare exceptions where the loss of emotional depth in dementia 'improves' someone's personality.) Our standards should be set not by our own ideas of cleanliness, activity, sociability, or intelligence but by the patient's previous standard. Thus an untidy person is not dementing just because her house is untidy; there must be evidence of a definite and gradual decline. On the other hand, the evidence of a change is very obvious in someone who previously *was* very tidy and obsessional.

Background information continues to be relevant in other ways throughout the illness. For the less severely impaired the past is an anchor of reality that they can cling to. For both patients and families, past relationships and attitudes determine their present reactions. For the more severely impaired, fragments of past interests, attitudes, habits, relationships emerge from time to time. For families and professionals, the past is a constant reminder that this patient is a person, with long experience behind her, not a child.

There is therefore no excuse for the old practice of refusing access by junior nursing or care staff to background information about their charges. This invites an impersonal, infant-ilizing approach and prevents stimulating interaction. If staff are to be able to talk with a dementing patient at all at a

human level, they need to be able to encourage reminiscence, remind her of past interests and important relationships and to help her to share her past experiences with
others.

The patient's history

A surprising amount of information about the past can come
from the patient herself. Older and more important memories
may be maintained late in dementia, partly because they have
been rehearsed so often over the years that they are very
fixed, and partly because the patient returns to these
memories when the present and recent past are fading. She
will be able to give us some idea about her childhood and
early family relationships, together with some glimpses of her
jobs, her marriage, her children. In the earliest stages she will
be able to give quite a full account of her life up to recent
times. But this information must always be checked, for
memories become incomplete, and time sequences muddled.
The generations of the family may get mixed up in her mind,
and recent memories get put too far in the past or vice versa.
However, these more or less muddled memories are
important in understanding how the patient reacts to her
illness. Do resentments about the past sour her judgement
of the present? Does pride in the past make her reluctant to
accept her present dependence on others?

The relative's history

We can obtain far more information from relatives about her
previous personality, attitudes, level of activity, interests,
social functioning and self-care. It is important to help the
relatives separate recent events from events that happened
before the dementia began (and since the beginning is vague
this is a difficult task). This information will provide clear
evidence of how much change has occurred. And this helps
in understanding what new problems the family is having to
cope with and so helps to explain their reactions.

Background information gives the essential baseline in
assessing what support the patient can expect from family and
friends, what interests and activities she might continue to
engage in, and what her living conditions are. A simple *list*

of the family, with an indication of how near they live, how often they visit and their commitment can be helpful. Alternatively, a *timetable* of regular visitors and activities in the patient's normal lifestyle shows what can reasonably be expected. More detailed investigation of the relationships in the family and the attitudes of family members (Ch. 7) is also required. We need to know whether a good supportive relationship has existed in the past or whether there was animosity or indifference.

Diagnosing dementia

Chapters 1 and 2 explain that we need to make clear diagnosis as early as possible so that we can move on to plan the help which the patient will need. We need to reassure those who are not suffering from dementia, organize a later reassessment for those where there is doubt, and treat those patients with reversible dementia, and those who have other illnesses that are masquerading as dementia (the pseudodementias).

We need to be particularly on the look out for 'dementia' that has a rapid onset and has one or more of the typical features of acute confusion (Table 2.4), for signs of depression (p. 57) and for hints of other physical illnesses. But we also need to remember that whilst these other illnesses may indeed be all that is wrong with the patient, there are many cases where there are two diagnoses — dementia and the other illness. For example, hypothyroidism can *cause* a dementia but many people with ATD or MID also suffer from hypothyroidism which is *not* worsening their mental state. In the former case thyroid replacement treatment will reverse the dementia, but in the latter treatment will leave the dementia unchanged.

So, if there is positive evidence for another diagnosis, that illness should be treated first and then the patient should be reassessed. But dementia itself should be diagnosed positively, as well as by excluding other illnesses. To make a proper diagnosis of dementia we need three bits of evidence:

1. There must be significant impairment of many brain functions
2. The impairments must be steadily progressive
3. Other diagnoses must be ruled out.

Detecting losses

Looking at the losses described in Chapter 4 we can see that much information can be got from interviewing and examining the patient and by observing her carrying out her daily tasks; by observing, in effect, how she 'uses her brain'. In interview it is possible to assess orientation, detect memory impairments and other intellectual loss, observe speech difficulties, and test special functions such as those of the parietal lobe.

The patient's appearance and behaviour give useful information about poor self-care, lost social skills, disinhibition and poor attention or concentration. Her attitude to the losses that are revealed is most important. Is she upset, or apathetic. Does she try to cover up (Table 6.2)? Are her emotions stable or labile? Does she have good insight? In the course of an interview, evidence that she has mistaken beliefs, or hallucinations can be obtained, though sometimes very direct questioning is required.

Rating scales. Some of the information about intellectual impairment is summarized in the standard intellectual rating scales (Table 9.2), but strictly speaking, these were not invented to make diagnosis, and are certainly not enough in themselves. Other deficits or illnesses may cause a person to perform poorly on these scales. So they can only be *part* of our assessment. The same argument applies to observations that are used in behaviour rating scales (Table 9.3). Both are better used to indicate *degree* of dementia or degree of *dependence*.

Showing progressive decline

All this information put together indicates what losses have occurred. But it must always be remembered that an interview or an observation represents how the patient is at one particular time; it must always be put in the perspective of the *course* of the changes.

Evidence from relatives. Relatives will be able to fill in many more details. But, more important, it is only the relatives who can give an account of the course of the illness. They will need guidance in giving their account. They will need to be reminded of the many areas of function that might be declining (see Ch. 4). And the criteria that there must be both a change and a continuing decline should be applied to each loss separately.

Because a particular close relative is likely to have strong feelings about the patient, or because the relative may not be with the patient all the time, it is often necessary to have more than one account. Other relatives, the sheltered house warden, the home help, friends and neighbours, shopkeepers, police, lawyers, clergy — all may have bits of information which complete the picture or correct a biased account of how the patient has deteriorated mentally.

In many cases the combination of a history from the patient and other informants with a god examination of the mental state of the patient and some observation of her behaviour will ensure a proper diagnosis of dementia.

Ruling out other causes

However, in some cases there are doubts that remain. These are cases of possible pseudodementia, cases of early dementia and cases where there is another potential diagnosis, e.g. a thyroid problem. A history of depression in the past, and of depressive symptoms beginning before the onset of the 'dementia' can help in diagnosing a pseudodementia. Interview and observation may hint that the correct diagnosis is depression rather than dementia. We might expect shrinkage of the brain to show up on a CT scan in a case of dementia, but not in a case of depression. But among elderly people there are many false positives (patients who do not have dementia but show shrinkage) and false negatives (those who do have dementia but no obvious shrinkage). In younger patients this is not the case and scans are an essential part of diagnosis.

Slowing of the regular rhythms of the electroencephalogram (EEG) and changes in the electrical activity of the temporal lobe are often found in dementia, so this can add to the certainty of diagnosis. Again this type of evidence is not very specific. A search is going on for tests which will distinguish dementia from pseudodementia, or from normality. For example, a development of the EEG, called the auditory evoked potential, may help. This adds together the tiny electrical brain responses that can be detected over the auditory cortex when a sound or light is repeated many times. In dementia, some parts of the response are delayed. At present this is not an accurate diagnostic test, but from this type of development, useful tests may eventually come. Newer developments in scanning, such as nuclear magnetic resonance (NMR) and positron emission tomography (PET) will offer more sophisticated pictures of brain damage, and in the case of PET, can show aspects of the activity of the brain, such as blood flow and the metabolism of essential chemicals. On the other side, accurate tests for depressive illness may eventually prove helpful. An early try is the dexamethasone suppression test which measures the effects of changes in steroid hormones that occur in many depressed people. However, this test is not specific enough to be helpful in diagnosis. The best evidence remains a proper, well researched history and examination.

In the last 10 years attempts have been made to develop elaborate questionnaires which will ensure proper diagnosis of dementia. Some of these have computerized versions which should help to ensure standardization in diagnosis. They are not for everyday use as yet. We need shorter versions of these tests which can both establish the diagnosis of dementia and rule out other possibilities.

Diagnosing dementia has momentous consequences for the patient and her family. As a wrong diagnosis is equally momentous, every patient deserves proper investigation to ensure that the diagnosis is accurate, and that other causes have been excluded. This means that all younger cases and most older cases should be referred to a geriatrician or psychogeriatrician as early as possible after the telltale changes begin. Unfortunately, older people often suffer an ageist negligence in this respect.

The type of dementia

The best test of which type of dementia a patient suffers from would be a brain biopsy, which involves taking a tiny sample of the patient's brain during life, by operation, and seeing the pathology of the dementia. However, because of the risks of the operation, the uncertain effects of biopsy on brain function and the fact that there is as yet no treatment for the common dementias, this test is rarely carried out. In deciding how far to go with tests that are currently available to differentiate the various types of dementia, we need to consider two age groups.

Patients who begin to dement over the age of 70

The older one is at the beginning of dementia, the less likely are the rarer and the reversible types of dementia relative to ATD and MID. ATD and MID increase in frequency with age. Some illnesses such as Huntington's chorea specifically affect younger people. So the most likely other diagnoses in an older person are normal pressure hydrocephalus and brain tumour, and these are quite uncommon. Thus the general feeling among specialists is that it is not worthwhile going to great lengths to find these conditions *unless* there are suggestive symptoms — for NPH, unexplained early incontinence, gait dyspraxia and a history of head injury etc. (p. 29); for a tumour, signs or symptoms of very local damage to an area of the brain out of proportion to the severity of the dementia ('localizing signs'), signs of raised fluid pressure within the skull due to the growth of the tumour within a confined space (raised intra-cranial pressure) or, since most brain tumours are secondary growths spread from primary tumours elsewhere in the body, evidence of a primary growth.

Other types of reversible dementia due to physical illnesses can be detected for more easily. The screening tests in Table 9.1 are therefore worth carrying out in all patients

Patients who begin to dement below 70

The chances of a diagnosis other than ATD or MID increase the younger the onset of the dementia. Since many of these other causes have some treatment, investigation is important. Everyone that is suspected to be suffering from dementia should have the screening tests mentioned above, and a CT or other scan test. It must be stressed that the fact that older patients are not quite so extensively investigated is not a sign of ageism. It is entirely justified by the relative incidence of the various treatable causes of dementia.

Table 9.1 Screening tests in the diagnosis of types of dementia

Test	Diagnosis
Full blood count and vitamin B12 and folate	Vitamin B12 deficiency Folate deficiency
VDRL and TPHA blood tests	General paralysis of the insane
Thyroid function tests	Hypothyroidism
Blood calcium and phosphorus	Parathyroid disorder
CT or NMR scan	Brain tumour Normal pressure hydrocephalus

ATD or MID?

How important is it to know which of the two common causes a patient (of any age) has? The only practical difference it makes is that we can warn the relatives of a different prognosis. In ATD we expect a slow gradual decline, with death probably occurring gently after a mild chest infection. In MID we cannot predict the course so well, but we can warn the relatives of possible sudden changes, periods of stability, patchy losses of function and the quite likely occurrence of other illnesses due to arteriosclerosis. Death is more likely to be sudden. It is not worth spending money on expensive and sometimes disturbing tests for this benefit. The Hachinski score (Table 1.8), using background information from relatives about other arteriosclerotic problems and present evidence of multiple small strokes, gives a rough diagnostic guide, though it is not entirely reliable. The CT scan, and more successfully, the NMR scan, can show strokes in the brain, but using these more expensive tests simply to tell ATD from MID is not justified. In any case many patients have both conditions at the same time (p. 27).

The severity of dementia

By severity of dementia, we should not mean how disturbed a patient is. In Chapters 5 and 6 we have seen that disturbed or disinhibited behaviour and the patient's emotional reactions may be at their height early in the dementia. If we want

Table 9.2 An intellectual rating scale — the Hodkinson Memory Information Scale (adapted from Hodkinson H M 1972 Age and Ageing 1:223)

1. What age are you?
2. What is the time?
3. Repeat back an address (42, West Street) and then try to recall it at the end of the test.
4. What year is it?
5. Name this place.
6. Recognize two people.
7. What date were you born?
8. What were the dates of the First World War?
9. What is the name of the present monarch?
10. Count backwards from 20 to 1.

Score 1 for each correct answer.

to measure the true severity, that is, how far the damage to the brain has gone, we need a general measure of the losses of function, ignoring disinhibition and reactions. It is very difficult to obtain a reliable measure. The usual behaviour rating scales, for example, contain questions that relate to disturbed behaviour.

Rating scales. It is information on the wide variety of losses which, added together, gives a real indication of severity. When we try to do this adding, we find however that, inevitably, some functions are more damaged than others. The losses of dementia do not occur in a uniform fashion in every patient, nor at the same rate for each loss. But it has been shown that asking a few questions from the mental state examination, usually about ten, can give a fairly good general indication of the level of impairment. This is an *intellectual rating scale* (Table 9.2). The lower the score, the more severely demented the patient is, always remembering that we should try to compare with the patient's own normal level of function.

Beyond a moderate level of dementia, patients are likely to score 0 or 1 on these tests for the rest of their life. So they are useful only in earlier stages when they can be very helpful in charting the *progress* of the dementia. If the patient's score gets better rather than worse, some further thought is required about the diagnosis.

Because of the limitations of intellectual rating scales, *behaviour rating scales* (Table 9.3) have been devised. Much

Table 9.3 A behaviour rating scale — the Modified Crichton Geriatric Behaviour Rating Scale (originally devised by R. A. Robinson)

Dimension		Score
Mobility	Fully ambulant including stairs	0
	Usually independent	1
	Walks with minimal supervision	2
	Walks only with physical assistance	3
	Bed-fast or chair-fast	4
Orientation	Complete	0
	Orientated in ward, identifies persons correctly	1
	Misidentifies persons but can find way about	2
	Cannot find way to bed or toilet without assistance	3
	Completely lost	4
Communication	Always clear, retains information	0
	Can indicate needs, understands simple verbal directions, can deal with simple information	1
	Understands simple information, cannot indicate needs	2
	Cannot understand information, retains some expressive ability	3
	No effective contact	4
Co-operation	Actively co-operative, i.e. initiates helpful activity	0
	Passively co-operative	1
	Requires frequent encouragement or persuasion	2
	Rejects assistance, shows independent but ill-directed activity	3
	Completely resistive or withdrawn	4
Restlessness	None	0
	Intermittent	1
	Persistent by day	2
	Persistent by day, with frequent nocturnal restlessness	3
	Constant	4
Dressing	Correct	0
	Imperfect but adequate	1
	Adequate with minimum supervision	2
	Inadequate unless continually supervised	3
	Unable to dress or retain clothing	4
Feeding	Correct, unaided at appropriate times	0
	Adequate, with minimum supervision	1
	Inadequate unless continually supervised	2
	Needs to be fed	3

Table 9.3 (*cont'd*)

Dimension		Score
Continence	Full control	0
	Occasional accidents	1
	Continent by day only if regularly toileted	2
	Urinary incontinence in spite of regular toileting	3
	Regular or frequent double incontinence	4

of the information on these scales refers to the losses of dementia and changes right through the later stages of dementia. It is important to extract this information if we wish to gauge the severity of the dementia, for the overall score on a behaviour scale indicates the severity *plus* disturbance of the patient. This overall score gives an indication of how much *help* she will need and so can predict the best *placement* for her, but it is wrong to use total scores of these scales as evidence of *severity*. Like intellectual scales, behaviour scales are best used to chart progress, particularly when attempts are being made to improve the patient's behaviour.

The value of knowing the severity of dementia is in any case limited. It tells us very roughly how dependent the patient is, and allows us to chart the decline. It can help to emphasize that a particular symptom (say incontinence) is occurring out of sequence in the decline, but only in a very general way. It is little help in telling what sort of care the patient ought to by receiving (p. 76). It gives no indication of how long the dementia will last.

Staging dementia. Table 9.4 shows one attempt to classify the stages of dementia. It is useful as a general guide to what we should call mild, moderate and severe, so that we all use the same language; people who are unused to dementia are likely to call a mild case 'severe'. But these stages are not rigid in any way and mean little for an individual patient, except as a very general guide and an indication of what should surprise if it happens in 'mild' rather than 'severe' patients.

Problems

In practice, once the diagnosis has been made we can best

Table 9.4 The stages of dementia (loosely based on Hughes C P et al 1982 British Journal of Psychiatry 140:566)

Healthy	No memory loss, orientated, solves problems, has outside interests, independent in home and in self-care.
Questionable dementia	Mild forgetfulness, but orientated, doubtful impairment of problem-solving and general interest outside and inside the home, independent in self-care.
Mild dementia	Moderate recent memory loss affecting daily life, some disorientation in time, may be disorientated in place in strange surroundings, difficulty handling any complex problems, cannot maintain outside interests, abandons complicated tasks at home, needs some prompting in self-care.
Moderate dementia	Severe memory loss, retains only highly learnt material, disorientated in time and often in place, cannot handle problems or make judgements, unable to function independently away from home, only does the simplest chores at home, needs some assistance in dressing, hygiene etc.
Severe dementia	Severe memory loss, fragmentary mental activity, completely disorientated except to own identity, unable to solve any problems or make judgements, unable to care for self or to function at home or outside, often incontinent.

approach dementia by looking at *problems*, rather than severity. It is these specific problems which burden relatives and require special attention and treatment, rather than the severity of the illness. This goes a long way to explaining why some mildly demented people are in hospitals and some severely demented are at home (p. 77).

We can only examine a patient's problems properly when we have made the diagnosis, got a full history, examined and observed her extensively, and know a considerable amount about her background. But right from the beginning, the list of problems will be emerging, for it is likely to be one specific problem which has brought the patient for help of whatever kind. It is unlikely that the main problem at the time of referral is simply the gradual decline, unless we have detected the patient by screening or case-finding.

The problem orientated approach

What is a *problem*? It is a title, in as few words as possible, one word best of all, which describes some aspects of the experience or behaviour of the patient, which she, her relatives or others around her find distressing or difficult to cope with. There will be many stories or anecdotes of what the patient feels or does. In working out a problem list, our aim is to simplify those stories into the smallest number of problem titles which will be comprehensive. We need to use two problem titles only when one will not suffice. If a patient wanders, and is unsteady on her feet when out wandering, then there are two problem titles — 'wandering' and 'unsteadiness' — even though the two things happen at the same time. If she wanders by day and by night but the consequences of both are the same, namely that she is at risk of being mugged, then there is one problem title. In practice it is up to each individual or team to decide how much they are going to join problems together and how much they separate them into smaller problems. However, for a general assessment I suggest that a list which contains somewhere between four and ten problems for a dementing patient is plenty to be both comprehensive and to plan for effective action. Table 9.5 shows a typical problem list.

Behaviour rating scales can be useful in working out what problems a patient has, because they can act as a checklist, but our full checklist of potential problems is endless (see Table 3.4). The purpose of the problem list is as a starting point for action, but it also describes the patient in a simple and effective way. It can, for example, be used in talking to relatives. After the relatives have given their account, the interviewer can feed back the list of problems they have been compiling, asking 'Does that sum up all the difficulties as you see them?'. Relatives can then feel that they have got their message across and that it is understood (or not) and have the opportunity to add extra details.

Causes of problems

Having formulated our problem list, the next step is to try to work out *why* the problem is occurring. This is *not* the time to rush into action. It is a time for thought and further assessment if needed. Chapters 4–7 have shown how to think about causes. We can indeed almost always explain the causes of

Table 9.5 A problem list for a day hospital patient

Name	Mrs. J. McK.
Date of birth	25 - 8 - 02
Address	15 Castle Grove
Date admitted	17 - 5 - 87
Proposed length of stay	Medium
Purpose(s) of attendance	Assessment and relief for relatives
Number of days attending	2
Family supports	Lives with daughter and family
Support services	Health visitor / Sitter service

Date	Problem	Action	By whom	Date of review	Outcome
5·87	Restlessness in house	Physical assessment	Doctor	6·87	Constipated
		Organised activity	Sitter and daughter OT	6·87	Slight improvement
		Treat constipation (6·87)	Doctor and nursing staff	7·87	Much improved Still some present
		Thioridazine 20 mg. (7·87)	GP	8·87	Much better
5·87	Sleep disturbance	More activity by day	as above	6·87	Improved
5·87	Bathing	Assessment	OT	6·87	Aids provided
5·87	Accuses daughter of stealing	Reassurance	Nursing staff	6·87	No better
		Thioridazine 20mg (7·87)	GP	8.87	Slightly better
5·87	Daughter depressed and anxious	Information booklet	Day hospital	5·87	
		See CPN	CPN	6·87	Little improvement
		Family meeting	All staff	7·87	For respite admission (8·87)

a problem under one or more of the headings of Loss, Disinhibition, Personal reaction and Family reaction (Table 9.7). As we have gone through these types of cause we have seen a number of examples (Tables 5.2, 6.1) of problems and their analysis. The importance of discovering the *different types of cause* is that they require *completely different management*.

Of course things are rarely simple in dementia. It is not always possible to define problems as clearly as we might like, the cause may be obscure or multiple, and the whole assessment is rather subjective — what one person sees as a problem, another may think is not worth bothering about. Group discussion of problems and their causes is the best system.

The value of a problem-orientated approach is that is leads logically to action if the cause or causes of the problem can be identified. The most pressing problem obviously must take precedence. We can quickly see how a crisis has arisen, and how to prevent a loss of independence if we describe *crucial* problems. 'If that problem was solved, the family could cope', for example. Some of the problems will be *inactive* rather than *active* ones, and some of the active ones may not need very urgent attention, but this comprehensive shorthand description of the patient is practical and easy to recall.

Problems not due to dementia

It is important to try to separate off any problems that are not due to dementia. There is a great temptation to lump everything that is wrong with the patient and blame it on her dementia. But other illnesses, loss of sight or hearing, mobility problems, drug side-effects, and family troubles may have nothing at all to do with it, though they will have an influence on the patient's management and treatment. They will not, however, follow the typical course of the problems of dementia itself.

METHODS OF ASSESSMENT

Talking to the patient

Some people seem to have the knack of talking with dementing people. Others have to learn it over time. Some, who probably were not interested anyway, never learn. In Chapters 4, 5 and 6 I have mentioned a number of important ways to compensate for the patient's losses in interview and ways to deal with disinhibition and the patient's reactions. Here I wish to bring together some general principles which can ease our assessment and help conversation generally.

1. Explain what is happening — introduce yourself and explain why you want to talk to the patient, in a way that she is likely to understand. Say what is going to happen in the interview. This information may well have to be repeated several times.

2. Find out how the patient feels about the interview — she may be unable to understand what is happening, or not wish to know; she may object, believing that she does not need help; she may think something completely different is happening. All these reactions affect the quality of information that we get.

3. Don't spend too long. Poor attention and fatigue can make the patient muddled or emotionally upset. Come back again later. Within the interview, intersperse questions or mental 'work' with general talk, reminiscence etc.

4. Allow for sight, hearing and speech problems. Help the patient who has expressive problems by guessing what she means; do not leave her to try desperately to get her message across.

5. For all patients, not only those with receptive dysphasia, use simple speech, not complicated sentences. This does not mean treating the patient like a child.

6. Use non-verbal communication. A smile, a friendly touch, a firm handshake can help the patient feel more at ease. Once again do not treat her like a child.

7. Go at the patient's pace. This will always be slower than our pace. The correct pace has to be worked out at the time. With severely demented people there may have to be long gaps and silences, and very few words need to be spoken.

8. Do not change the subject too quickly. Remember perseveration, the difficulty in moving from one subject to another.

9. Repeat messages, not in a way that puts the patient under pressure, but in a way that helps the message get

across. Saying the same thing in differing ways may help. Cues help her to get more answers.

10. Expect and look for emotional changes in the interview. If a particular line of questions is upsetting, take the pressure off, sympathize with her feeling and then change the subject for a while.

11. Allow for any disinhibited reactions of inexplicable tears, laughter, anger, over-affection, or the catastrophic reaction. Again give the patient a rest. The interviewer should never respond spontaneously to such reactions. If the patient finds her reaction distressing, reassurance is needed.

12. It can be useful, however, to find out how she does cope under pressure by asking a quick series of questions or changing the subject quickly. This can give an estimate of how she would cope at home if something went wrong, if someone was trying to exploit her, or if she was in a strange situation.

13. Talking to a dementing person should seem natural and relaxed *to her*. We need to be flexible and modify our approach, depending on her personality and what she expects. Some patients prefer a formal approach, others less formal. Some cope with physical contact more than others, some appreciate more sympathy than others. We will get more information if the patient feels that we are on her side.

14. Information from interviews does not come in an orderly sequence. We may have interviewed the patient to help diagnosis, assess problems, discuss plans of management or talk of going into care. As far as possible we should try to stick to the purpose of the interview. But other things are going on which will tell us of speech problems, how the patient is feeling, about family relationships, attitudes, or completely new difficulties that we had not known of. Always keep an open mind and an observant eye. Review what has been learnt afterwards.

15. End on a positive and friendly note, even if some of the interview has been upsetting. Summarize simply what has been said so that she can have some memory of what went on. If the summary is upsetting, end with general conversation and then a formal farewell, preferably with a handshake.

16. Do not base judgements on one interview. The patient

may perform very differently in other settings or at other times. Find out about these other times.

Talking with relatives

I have emphasized that family members have as much as or more information to offer than the patient. Indeed the problem usually is that they have too much to say. It is most important, therefore, to decide what is required from a family interview beforehand by preparing an *agenda*. The interviewer then has the task of ensuring that all the items of the agenda are discussed in the time available. Inevitably the relatives will want to introduce other subjects, and some of these have to be put to one side for discussion at another time. But what the relatives want to talk about is important to them. It may be that they have come to the interview with one message, or one strong feeling ('She can't stay at home any longer.' 'We are anxious about her safety.'). If these strong messages are not listened to and acknowledged, the family will feel dissatisfied and may not co-operate in giving information or agreeing to plans.

Therefore in proceeding with an interview, the interviewer should be aware not only of the agenda that *he* has brought along, but of the *relatives'* agenda. The interviewer should make sure that he understands these feelings and messages and should say so clearly. There may have to be a compromise between the two agendas.

In making an 'agenda' the problem-orientated approach works best. This allows discussion to fall under a number of headings. It also allows other problems to be raised at the end. If the interviewer is skilful, there will not be much that has been left out. The problem list is very helpful also for further meetings. Progress on each problem and the action taken can be discussed separately and efficiently.

While talking with relatives it is important to realize that they bring along feelings which are inevitably stronger than those of the interviewer and these feelings may bias or cloud their judgement. Part of the interviewer's job is to empathize or 'be with' those feelings but not to let *his* judgement be clouded or *his* decisions biased. The interviewer has to keep the reality of the situation, the patient's views, the professional assessments clearly in mind. The relatives' feelings are another factor, indeed one of the most important, but not the only one to be considered in making decisions.

We should also be on the lookout for gaps in education and knowledge of services which make it difficult for the family to come to wise decisions. Some part of most interviews will be spent in filling these gaps. The most important knowledge families must have is that their relative suffers from dementia and that this is progressive. As soon as it is possible to be sure about this, the family should be told. We can hope that then, after the initial shock, staff and family will be able to work on the same wavelength.

The relatives also need to know why all the information we ask for is necessary. They need an explanation of the importance of a baseline, and the necessity of identifying problems and looking for their causes if we are to help the patient effectively.

Families are not, however, simple organizations. In making a list of the family and their involvement (p. 253), the relationships in the family should become apparent. Some families have a head or spokesman and the rest will agree with his judgement. But most are much more diffuse, so that talking to one member is not sufficient. We should beware of false spokesmen who want their view to prevail in the family. We should be particularly aware of quieter members who may not be getting their views across. We are often dealing with several generations — the patient's brothers or sisters, spouse, children, grandchildren or great-grandchildren and in-laws. All their varying needs must be considered in working out what 'the family' feels.

Relatives and patient

In talking to relatives we should be continually aware that the patient is the patient. Her permission should always be asked before seeing them, and we should explain to her the reasons for wanting to see them.

Some relatives are happy to talk with the sufferer present, others find this very difficult. We should encourage openness between relative and patient, unless it is causing major distress to either. If, however, a relative refuses to talk with the patient present, ask why this is, but go along with the request for a private talk (after asking the patient's permission), for such a relative will be unlikely to give the whole story otherwise. Indeed it is useful to offer the opportunity of even a short private word with the relative, for there may be just one or two things which they feel unable to say in the sufferer's hearing.

It is sometimes tempting to listen only to the relative's story. Instead it can be very useful to use the information we get from them to ask more questions of the patient, about her background, her relationships, her present feelings. The result is a better understanding of both relatives and patient.

Observing the patient

Informal observation

Much useful information is gained by merely observing how a patient spends her time. Does she engage in activities or sit quietly? Are her activities purposeful or meaningless? Can she concentrate and persist in activity? Is she easily distracted? How much does she talk to other people and is she talking sense? Is she restless? Does she seem happy or otherwise? Is there any odd behaviour? All these can help in assessing the severity of dementia, show changes in the patient's state, indicate problems and suggest solutions.

Activities of daily living (ADL)

It is often more helpful to look more specifically at the things that everybody needs to do to manage from day to day. These include dressing and undressing (including remembering to change clothes), washing and bathing, toileting, eating, shopping for and cooking food, heating the house correctly, coping with laundry, dealing with bills, going to bed and sleeping. Many different losses of dementia can affect the patient's performance in these areas. They show up the practical effects of dementia. Impairments in these functions are more crucial to the patient's independent survival than whether she can recall a name and address. They will therefore be high on our problem list. Accurate and specialized assessment of daily living tasks is required. This is the special responsibility of the occupational therapist, as well as being part of the wider job of nursing and care staff. A few important points need to be made in relation to such assessments.

1. Remember the baseline. If people vary a great deal in their intelligence and interests, they vary even more in their standards of hygiene, pattern of daily living, styles of cooking and shopping. The standard for judging the patient's performance is her own, not ours.

2. Assess what she *needs* to be able to do *now*. The amount of independence in self-care that is needed by a dementing person varies depending on who she is, but also on her situation. A dementing man with a willing wife at home may get away with quite severe impairments in self-care without the wife feeling that the burden is too great. Unfortunately the opposite is not always the case. A patient who lives alone and refuses help needs all her daily living skills if she is to survive. To survive in residential care only a few basic skills of dressing, washing and toileting are required, and many get away with less.

3. Assessment should take place in the patient's home if possible. Many of our abilities in daily tasks are based on routines with familiar objects and equipment. Although it is useful to see how a patient deals with new equipment or a new environment (and this can be important if she is to move from her old home), testing in a special 'ADL suite' does not always give an accurate indication of how she would cope at home. There is no substitute for a visit home. If a patient has been in care for more than a few days, the return home may be difficult for she may be confused by the move, or have quickly got out of practice. More than one visit may therefore be required in order to make an accurate assessment.

4. Assessment should not be like a 'test'. Inevitably there is pressure on the patient to perform well and inevitably the person assessing is an 'intruder' in her home. But the skill of the assessor lies in making the situation feel as natural as possible to the patient. Acting like a friendly visitor, avoiding standing over the patient, not giving too many instructions, avoiding hurry and ensuring that the activities are done as nearly as possible to the way the patient would normally do them, can all be of help. Positive encouragement and praise

without pressure is helpful, so that she is able to relax and enjoy what she is doing.

5. As with interviews, it may nevertheless be useful once or twice to test the effects of pressure or hurry. For some patients, it is only when they are under pressure or things do not go along their usual routine that they make mistakes and get muddled.

6. In carrying out ADL assessments, the *purpose* should always be kept in mind. The assessment should lead to action. The action may be to improve the safety of the home, to recommend aids, to retrain the patient, to suggest ways in which the family could fill gaps, or to come to a decision about whether the patient can stay at home.

A proper ADL assessment requires a good knowledge of the particular patient, of possible aids and adjustments in the home and especially of the deficits that lead to practical difficulties. Understanding of sight, hearing and smell disorders, mobility problems, memory problems, agnosia, spatial problems, dyspraxia, attention problems, poor motivation, emotional lability are all needed, and useful information about all these types of deficit can be fed back to other staff who care for the patient as well as to the family.

Table 9.6 shows one example of an ADL assessment form.

Table 9.6 Information to be obtained from a home assessment, including activities of daily living

Description of accommodation		Access, including stairs
		General care of house, including warmth
		Rooms and equipment
		kitchen, bathroom, toilet,
		living room, bedrooms
		Heating and lighting
		Telephone, alarm system
Supports	Informal	Alone or not
		Visiting family, friends and neighbours
	Formal	Home help
		Sitting service
		Meals on wheels
		Laundry service
		District nurse
		Health visitor, CPN
		Social worker
		General practitioner

Outings	Shopping, pension, other regular outings
	Lunch club
	Day care

Timetable of regular visitors and outings

Mobility	Standing, walking, stairs
	Getting in and out of chair, bed, bath and on and off toilet
	Orientation in house
	Aids used
Other physical disabilities	Sight, hearing, smell
	Physical symptoms or signs
Personal care	General appearance and interest
	Dressing and undressing
	Washing and grooming
	Bathing or showering
	Toileting, including incontinence
	Reminders needed
	Aids used
Food preparation	Planning
	Shopping
	Food in store
	Assessment of making tea, a snack and a full meal
	Safety with kettle and cooker
	Eating
Household chores	Dishes
	Dusting and cleaning
	Laundry
Managing finances	Pension, bank
	Shopping
	Bills, rent etc.
	Money in the house
	Help with finances
Managing medication	Need for reminders
	Accuracy
Mental state during visit	Attention and concentration
	Restlessness
	Abnormal behaviour
	Orientation in time, place and person
	Communication
	Memory
	Agnosias and dyspraxia
	Emotions and motivation
	Abnormal beliefs
	Insight

This comprehensive look at the patient's abilities can be of the greatest value in determining what help is needed and where the patient can be. As with interviewing, it is vital however that one ADL assessment should not be used as the sole evidence of how the patient is coping. She may behave differently at different times or with different people. If the ADL assessment does not fit with other evidence, then both should be questioned.

Psychological testing

In the past it was customary for clinical psychologists to be involved in tests of intellectual capacity, learning and memory to make the diagnosis of dementia. Nowadays it is realized that as the general rule the mental state examination is effective enough to help in diagnosis and that special tests have not much to add. They still occasionally have their uses in diagnosis and assessment.

The tests which psychologists use include standard intelligence tests, and some modified ones, memory tests, tests of the ability to learn new material, tests of parietal lobe function (p. 95), reaction times. So they are of more use in defining specific areas of brain damage than in making the overall diagnosis. They may be useful, for example, when a patient is not doing as well as might be expected with a particular activity.

The development of computerized testing may alter the position of psychological testing. Using a simple push button or lever response, computer programmes have been devised which include elements of intelligence testing, the ability to learn new material, speed tests and memory. Eventually these tests will be of value in the early detection of dementia, for they are easier to standardize and take away the influence of the tester on the results. But like every method, the results have to be interpreted sensibly and in context. They only tell how the patient performs at that time and not at another time of day or in another situation. Such techniques will not be useful for later stages of dementia. We have also to remember that the next generation of elderly people, as well as the present one, will not be able to handle any more complicated computer material.

Rating scales

There are two types of rating scales in regular use — the intellectual (Table 9.2) and the behavioural (Table 9.3). As we have seen, these scales have been overused in diagnosis, and have a limited value in identifying problems. They are most informative when used to measure the progression of impairments over time and to predict the future care needs of the patient. They should not however be a lazy person's substitute for good history-taking, intelligent observation and full mental testing, which alone can show the vast range of deficits and disturbances caused by dementia.

In using the rating scales, some points are worth remembering:

1. Decide what the scale is to be used for before using it. What action will follow from its results? Routine testing of everybody in a ward, home or in day care might be useful for research purposes, but is unlikely to be useful in practice.

2. Decide how often it needs to be used in order to show up the changes that are being measured.

3. Try to standardize the use of the scales by having practice sessions with all staff involved.

4. Try to ensure that the information is accurate, not just hearsay or one individual's biased report. The use of rating scales should help improve the sharpness of observation and testing rather than lead to sloppiness.

5. Try to ensure that the information is valid for the whole day, not just the good times or the bad times. The difficulty of getting accurate and reliable information for rating scales reminds us just how variable a dementing person's performance can be.

6. Interpret the results intelligently. Remember how physical illness and drugs (p. 44) as well as poor attention, poor hearing, dysphasias, restlessness and poor motivation can interfere with intellectual testing; how losses interact (p. 91); and how loss of control can produce contrary effects (e.g. emotions, p. 135). No rating scale tells *why* the patient acts in one particular way. That question must be asked, but must be asked separately.

7. Remember that total scores only give a very general guide to the level of impairment or dependence. Look closely

at individual scores and the changes that occur in them. Then rating scales can help enormously in the day-to-day care of dementia sufferers.

In theory it might be better if we could devise individual ratings for each of the problems of each patient. But the popular rating scales offer a useful shorthand way of recording some of the commonest problems of dementia.

Medical examination

It has already been pointed out (p. 47) that the dementing patient is often unable to give a good account of the physical complaints of any illness. Even severe pain may be forgotten quickly or not described clearly. We have seen that acute confusion, emotional distress or restlessness may be the only signs that the patient is ill. Every dementing patient, therefore, deserves a regular (though not very frequent) medical check.

Medical examination is also necessary at the time of diagnosis, to exclude other causes of apparent impairment, to determine the cause of the dementia, and to look for quite separate physical illnesses. A medical check is also called for if there is a sudden change in the patient's condition, or if one of the symptoms or signs that develop does not fit into the usual pattern of dementia.

Obviously there is special emphasis on neurological examination, and this is particularly difficult in dementing patients because much of it depends on carrying out orders — 'move your leg', 'touch your nose' — and on reporting sensations — 'did you see that', 'did you feel that'. Particularly in MID there will, however, be widespread neurological damage. Often strokes have very minor or no observable neurological effects or they have unusual or mixed effects. General physicians need reminded of these facts. It is far too easy to say that a stroke has not occurred just because there is no paralysis or other physical signs. Yet both the stepwise and the gradual changes of MID are due to a series of hundreds of separate stroke events.

The doctor needs to be particularly painstaking in examining dementing patients, for he will not have the guidance of a good history from the patient. And in older patients there may of course be several different diagnoses. The time is worth spending, however. It is remarkable, for example, how often a rectal examination reveals constipation as the cause of restlessness. It is also remarkable how many illnesses are neglected for many months by patients, and even by their families, who may think the symptoms or signs are part of the dementia, or 'just old age'.

Special tests

The arguments which justify good diagnostic examination and routine physical check-ups for dementia sufferers also justify the use of the special tests in Table 9.3. All these tests will lead to clear and useful action either in trying to reverse a dementia, or treating associated illnesses.

In choosing tests and interpreting them, we should note:

1. It saves time, energy and expense to realize that, since many older people have multiple medical problems, some or all of the investigations may have been carried out by another doctor. A little detective work can help enormously.

2. We should take into account how disturbing each test may be to the patient. Simple blood tests are a temporary nuisance only, whereas urine testing requires a little co-operation and is of course difficult in an incontinent patient. The more time and co-operation required for a test the more difficult it will be for the patient and the more we should question its necessity. A good CT scan or EEG test both require that the patient keeps quite still for up to 15 minutes; NMR scanning requires longer.

3. It is important to know that the normal values of several of these tests change as people grow older.

4. Some tests are more expensive than others. In particular a PET scanning facility costs several million pounds and this technique will only be available for research purposes and in one or two places. All the more usual tests of dementia, if justifiable for proper diagnosis or care, are worth the expense.

5. For several tests I have emphasized the problem of 'false positive' and 'false negative' results (see, for example, p. 255).

A diagnostic test is only justified if it is likely to give a conclusive result. However a combination of tests may increase the confidence of our diagnosis.

New tests

It remains difficult to be sure of the diagnosis of any dementia very early in its course. Indeed, we cannot be absolutely sure of the diagnosis until post-mortem in most cases. There is therefore a great need for tests that can be used during life. The evoked potential test has suggested one way forward. Changes in the levels of certain hormones in the blood which occur in ATD, and are thought to be related to the transmitter changes in the brain, suggest another. The best of all, brain biopsy, cannot be justified in the absence of effective treatments for MID or ATD. This area is one where great development is likely to happen in the next few years.

MANAGEMENT OF DEMENTIA

In the 'management' column of Table 9.7, I have summarized the various approaches which I have discussed fully in previous chapters. A little more needs to be said about curative treatments, and some comments are needed on the carrying out of management plans.

Reversing dementia

In Table 1.5 I listed the causes of treatable dementia. These are conditions in which treatment will change a case of dementia into one of brain damage. If the damage has not been severe, the patient has a good chance of regaining a reasonable level of function. It should go without saying that all patients with treatable dementias deserve that treatment and therefore deserve proper investigation. Although investigations are likely to be more extensive in a younger patient the age of the patient does not matter as far as treatment is concerned.

The main purpose of research into Alzheimer-type dementia and multi-infarct dementia is to move them into the group of treatable dementias.

Table 9.7 The causes of problems in dementia and possible styles of management

Cause	Management
Decline in function	Encourage the use of remaining function Fill gaps Retrain
Disinhibition	Behaviour management Encourage what is normal External control Drug treatment
Reactions to the experience of dementia	Listening with empathy Counselling and reassuring support Drug treatment
Reactions of relatives	Education Universality Support Counselling Respite from caring
Decision-making	Conference on rights and risks Patient keeps control Advocacy on patient's behalf Hand-over by patient Compulsory take-over of decisions
Physical disability, physical illness, acute confusion	Ensure proper medical investigation, treatment and rehabilitation Nursing care when necessary

Alzheimer-type dementia

There are four possible approaches to treatment:

1. The damaged brain could be encouraged to function more effectively. We have discussed, in dealing with the losses of dementia, external aids to fill memory and other gaps, stimulation of abilities that the patient has not been using and retraining. But there is no evidence as yet of any technique which will reverse the decline of dementia and bring lost faculties back. We can encourage a patient to use her failing memory in the most effective way possible, but still not actually improve her basic memory function.

2. Damaged connections might be encouraged to grow again. If ATD is due largely to a loss of connections between nerve cells, there might eventually be a drug treatment which

could reverse that process. There is even some evidence that a very stimulating environment can help nerves connect with each other, but how much this might help the actual functioning of the brain is unclear. There is little chance of a treatment which could make dead nerve cells grow again. For this reason it will be important to find early cases and treat them.

3. The lost neurotransmitters might be replaced. This has been tried by giving patients choline, but so far not with very encouraging results. Perhaps this type of treatment will work better in the old-old variety of ATD who have a purer acetylcholine loss. But the fact that other transmitters are involved, especially in younger patients, makes this approach to treatment less likely to succeed.

4. Whatever is causing the damage could be attacked. If, for example, it was aluminium or another metal poison, the levels of aluminium reaching the brain could be reduced. If it is a more complex form of chemical damage, then more complicated treatments might be necessary. Viral or other infectious causes are still being investigated.

When a treatment is available, and it surely is a 'when' rather than an 'if', it cannot be expected to reverse major brain damage. The most important task will then be to learn how to detect cases at the earliest stages to prevent worsening. And, except in the fourth type of treatment, the damage may still go on occurring, but delayed perhaps by a year or two. Such treatments would nevertheless transform the lives of dementia sufferers. They will raise interesting ethical issues for the future.

Multi-infarct dementia

The most effective treatment in MID would be prevention. As MID is related to arteriosclerosis and hypertension it can be hoped that dietary and other changes which are aimed at reducing the incidence of these conditions would also have an impact on dementia. A more specific preventative treatment is the use of drugs which reduce clot formation by affecting the blood platelets which are involved in the steps that lead to clotting. Drugs such as aspirin and dipyridamole have been used in this way and shown to have some useful effect. Most strokes are due to clotting or small emboli, though some are caused by bleeding from blood vessels, and multi-infarct dementia implies the occurrence of many, many small strokes. It remains to be seen whether these or similar drugs will prevent the deterioration of MID.

A wide variety of drugs has been used in attempts to improve blood flow to the brain in MID. These are unlikely to be effective because the reduction in blood flow happens as a *result* of the brain damage or underuse and not as a *cause* of it. So increasing blood flow would not improve function.

A number of so-called 'cerebral activators' have also been used. It is not always clear what such drugs are supposed to do, and drug trials show varied or equivocal results. It is safest to assume that there is, as yet, no drug which has proved effective in improving the function of the damaged brain in either MID or ATD.

Carrying through management plans

My aim in this book has been to show that, despite the lack of curative treatments, we can approach the care and treatment of dementing people rationally with some hopes of alleviating the problems experienced by sufferers and their families. Each of Chapters 4–8 has described specific ways of managing the wide variety of problems. If such managements are to be effective in lessening distress and improving the quality of life of patients and relatives, a few general principles need to be applied.

1. Set reasonable goals

What is reasonable must be judged by reference to the pre-illness situation and our assessment of the present deficits and changes.

The further away from her normal the patient has moved, the more unlikely does it become that she will be able to get back to normal. Thus although we should always refer back to her previous life as a baseline, yet we should not raise our hopes and those of her family unnecessarily. Remember that none of the techniques described in Chapter 4 will replace lost functions. Only occasionally will retraining have any impact at all. Otherwise we can only try to fill gaps from outside, keep encouraging the patient to use her abilities to the full, and help her cope with the losses. We can hope to have some impact on disinhibitory symptoms and emotional reactions, but even here I have emphasized the limitations of treatment. Furthermore we have seen many examples of how losses and other problems interact and make helping more difficult. Over-optimism leads to disappointment just as under-optimism leads to poor morale.

2. Establish priorities

Since every patients has multiple problems we could invent a long list of possible management programmes in every case. What we actually choose to do should be guided by deciding what are the crucial problems (p. 265), what are the biggest problems, which cause most distress to the patient or her family, which are the easiest to treat. From this we should be able to make a list of priorities and start working down that list. Attempting too many treatments at once can be confusing, for it may be impossible to know which has helped. So relatives may have to be warned that we will be trying to deal with only one or two problems at a time. We will all need considerable patience.

3. Decide who is to carry out the management

There is not much use in assessing problems and formulating elaborate management plans if no-one is prepared to do the donkey work of actual management. Team or conference decision-making can help the fair sharing of work. As we shall see in Chapter 10, only certain jobs are anybody's specific responsibility in dementia; many jobs can be carried out by any one of a number of workers. Enthusiasm and willingness usually have to be complemented with patience if any of these techniques are to work. If a person is delegating to another worker or teaching the family how to help, he has a responsibility to continue to support the worker or family and to inject his own energy and enthusiasm into the programme. This is particularly true of group activities, slow retraining, reality orientation and behavioural programmes.

4. Call in expert help where necessary

As there are so many different types of problem in dementia it is most unlikely that one person, or even one team can manage all aspects of the care of a patient. We should never be ashamed to have to ask for an expert assessment or for expert help in management. Of course we can hope that the expert will teach us something that we can use again in the future, but no-one is an expert in everything. So the primary care team should call the psychogeriatric or geriatric service in early, residential homes should have no hesitation in calling expert nursing, physiotherapy, speech therapy or medical help, hospital teams may need the advice of other specialists, and should ensure that they are not ignoring the expertise that exists in the community.

5. Tell the patient what is happening

A dementing person may not be able to understand fully what is happening round about her. But she will have difficulty coping with changes, new faces, and new styles of treatment. As far as possible, we should explain to her what we propose to do, and why. There is no excuse for ignoring her.

6. Engage the family in treatment plans

They not only need to be told what our plans are, but are often important members of the treatment team. We have seen this particularly in relation to managing behaviour problems. But they also need to be taught gap-filling techniques, told how best to cope with emotional disturbances, and how to deal practically with physical problems such as incontinence, immobility, dressing problems and fits. They must learn the side-effects of the drugs they are supervising, and many other respects of management. Continuing contact and co-operation with the family throughout is therefore essential.

7. Set a time scale

Treatment plans should not drift on without reassessment. For each problem that is being assessed we should have a rough idea of how long the management will take, so that whoever is taking on the job can plan ahead, and so that a date for reassessment can be set.

8. Record what is decided

A problem sheet such as Table 9.5 (there are other variants of this) allows an accurate record of decisions, reminds people of the responsibilities they have taken on and allows clear reassessment.

9. Assess success or failure

When the time for review comes, or when difficulties occur in the programme, the status of the problem should be reassessed. If the goals are not reached, the problem needs to be reassessed and, if possible, a different strategy tried. Failure can be due to a mistaken assessment of the problem, over-optimistic (or under-optimistic) goals, imperfect carrying out of the programme, or a change in the whole situation (a further decline in the patient, for example) as well as all sorts of extraneous factors. The reasons for failures need to be recorded under 'outcome'. This leads on to a reformulation of the management plan.

CONCLUSION

Problem-orientated working is simple to organzie. It requires that the people involved sit down together regularly to plan and reassess the patient's care. There are many advantages in using proper multi-disciplinary team work. It leads to good communication between professions and with families, and wider education about the variety of management techniques available. A patient who is dealt with by one or two people in isolation misses out on a lot of the possibilities for help.

But often, the possibilities of helping are not as available as they should be. It would be difficult to make all the conceivable environmental changes necessary to improve a patient's comfort, safety and better orientation. It is difficult for hard pressed staff to spend the time they might wish to support relatives, or to keep patients engaged in activities. So management often has to be rationed. And while this is so there is still a 'political' task of ensuring that resources of money, people and places are available to help in the proper management that dementing patients deserve. In the meantime we have to provide care as comprehensively as we can with the resources available, focusing on the worst problems, using family as staff, setting realistic goals, giving treatment in groups where possible.

Nevertheless, the whole problem-orientated approach can transform the attitudes of those working with dementing people from a pessimistic despair to an optimistic but realistic commitment. For at all stages of the decline, it shows how 'success' that is limited, but no less real for that, can be achieved, even if the outcome always includes decline and eventual death.

10

Organizing help

As we have examined the many and changing problems of dementia, we have seen a variety of ways of helping. As dementia is a disorder which has a multitude of effects on the patient and her family, organizing help can be a complicated matter. In this chapter we shall look at the organizations involved and then at the different professional groups and their responsibilities before looking at how co-ordination of care and planning could be improved.

Defining responsibilities

Core. Each profession or organization will attempt to define its role in relation to an illness like dementia. But as we try to define our individual roles we can see that there are some responsibilities that are clear, some not so clear. The clearest of these make up the 'core' of our responsibility.

Thus doctors are the only people who can write a prescription, and they have special training in diagnosis and special access to facilities which help in diagnosis. Social workers have specific roles in arranging admission to residential homes and in relation to the Mental Health Act (p. 236).

District nurses have special training and responsibility in carrying out nursing tasks in the patient's own home.

Overlap. But a professional who tried to keep only to the core of his job would have a narrow and unsatisfied life. He would have to spend much of his energy in passing patients on to other professionals. To work together we must accept considerable *overlapping* of roles. Many tasks can be handled by any one of a variety of groups.

Mutual advice. Between these two types of responsibility, the core and the overlapping, there are areas where one professional will be able to *advise* another how to do a job which is close to his own core responsibility. Thus a physiotherapist will help nursing staff in techniques of lifting and in passive and active exercising. A clinical psychologist may teach staff in a home how to keep a behavioural chart. A community psychiatric nurse may teach a home help to look out for particular side-effects of drugs. Families may be taught by a variety of professionals to become 'amateur therapists'.

Job satisfaction. It could be said that professionals tend to feel satisfied in their work if they feel that they have clear responsibilities in their core job and that others respect that core without trying to tell them how to do their work; if they can freely overlap with others in the more general aspects of helping, not keeping exclusively to their core, but avoiding rivalry over who does what in these shared ares; and if they can pass on their skill and knowledge to others without meeting a hostile reaction. Of course there are some who prefer the overlapped areas of work, or even someone else's core to their own core responsibility! They are, as it were, in the wrong job, and it is up to others who work with them to decide how to react to this.

In a team the proper sharing of work between different professions depends on balances between the different cores and a fair division of labour.

Institutional responsibility

Institutions can be seen in a somewhat similar way. Each has a core responsibility for a particular type of dementing patient, but also accepts, and has to accept overlapping areas of responsibility for people who do not fit neatly into a 'Part III' category or a 'hospital' category. The staff of institutions can readily feel imposed upon if they have to look after more of the overlap patients than they themselves feel they should be coping with. And sometimes, of course, there are differing views from inside and outside about what an institution's responsibility should be.

For example, Part III homes see themselves as looking after only mildly demented people, or continuing to care for people as they dement further, as long as they are not too disturbed. Inevitably, they are taking far more of the severely demented population and keeping some who they think should be in hospital. Many local authorities are facing up to these problems, and are considering how they should adjust to accommodate the 'rising tide' of dementia sufferers. In the meantime there is limited job satisfaction for those who stick to the old ideas of their responsibility.

ORGANIZATIONS INVOLVED IN DEMENTIA

Let us look at each of the different organizations and see where their responsibilities lie.

The family

I have emphasized previously both the difficulties that face families and the ways in which they can be active in managing the problems of dementia. Family members learn from their own experience not only how to cope with their feelings about the illness, but how to cope practically with memory impairments by inventing memory aids, with restlessness by engaging the patient in useful activity, with poor self-care by filling gaps. Altogether they become quite as skilled as many professionals.

Apart from dealing with their own feelings and the change in relationship with the sufferer, carers have no role that is specifically laid down as their 'job'. What they take on in the way of care is entirely their own choice, and in this they differ from all the professions. Naturally, we expect the family to show loyalty and a continued wish to care, but we cannot insist on this. Furthermore, it is tempting for the professions to be so relieved when families cope with the less pleasant aspects of dementia that we let them get on with it. We should guard against letting families take on unreasonable burdens.

Sharing care

The family overlaps in its role with the roles of outside helpers and can therfore be seen as part of the treatment team. The inevitable conclusion is that the family should be involved in all decisions about how the work of caring is to be divided. In the same way, if they are discussing the division of labour among themselves, it is helpful if they bring professionals into the discussions. A family can also see *itself* as a team, and share the responsibilities between themselves like a professional team.

Thus working together and negotiating responsibilities allows better planning of care and avoids a sudden decision to abdicate responsibility for no reason. If the family members feel that their responsibilities are too much for them they should be perfectly at liberty to renegotiate their roles.

Financial help for carers

Families need more than just the recognition of outsiders to enable them to continue in their job of coping. There are expenses in caring and there may be loss of income if a relative has to give up work. *Attendance allowance* should be granted for any patient who requires regular care, though strangely this allowance is in theory given to the patient, so the assessor can sometimes be misled by a patient into thinking that she gets and requires no help. An appeal should correct this. *Invalid care allowance* and other benefits can also help. But all of this is small compared to the money spent on institutional care. In one or two areas DHSS funding, which would otherwise have gone to fund private residential care, has been available for families to buy appropriate care at home. This type of development brings the hope that the

work that many families do will be better supported finan-
cially in the future.

In Chapter 3 I emphasized changes in family structure
which will slowly lessen the number of fit relatives available
to help dementia sufferers directly. Planners will have to take
this into account in estimating how many families will be able
to cope and how many patients can stay 'in the community'.

The 'community'

This nebulous or non-existent body is believed in some quar-
ters to have an increasingly important role. In practice the
community usually means the family, or more precisely the
female members of the family, supported to a greater or
lesser extent by the primary care team and the home help
service. Gradually, however, voluntary organizations with a
special interest in dementia are developing. There are also
informal community supports which largely go unrecognized.
Friends and neighbours of a solitary dementing lady may play
a major role in her care, by checking that she is safe, by
helping with shopping or meals, even sometimes with more
intimate aspects of care. If they are heavily involved they
deserve recognition just as families do, by the respect of
professionals and with attendance allowance if appropriate.

The shopkeeper who keeps a dementing lady's money right
for her, or prevents her from repeatedly buying the same
thing is also involved in care, as is the policeman who gently
brings a wandering lady back home. They should all be in
communication with the more formal carers, so that everybody learns what the true situation is. Churches have a
special role to play in visiting, stimulating, providing meetings
and clubs. Unfortunately, some churches do not maintain
their loyalty to old members, who may have stopped
attending some years previously, or fallen out over a new
clergyman or unfamiliar music. Neighbourhood warden and
other 'checking-up' schemes are more formal and reliable
forms of community supervision for dementing people at
home.

The informal and voluntary network of care is very
important, but we cannot expect the amount of care offered
informally to increase greatly as the numbers of dementing

people increase in the community. So, if there is to be a shift from institutional forms of care to more care 'in the community', families and other informal carers who are already stretched to the limit will have to be relieved to a much greater extent by well organized voluntary or professional community supports.

The primary care team

The primary health care team of general practitioner, health visitor and district nurse, sometimes with other professionals, has a number of responsibilities throughout the course of dementia.

They should be involved in case-finding and accurate diagnosis, in planning care in liaison with family, social services and hospital services, in the support of families, and in the provision of medical and nursing care for patients who live at home.

Because of the balance of care (Table 3.5) the primary care team may be put in a position where alternatives to home care by the family are not available. Due to lack of understanding of dementia, or a feeling that it is 'just old age', general practitioners or health visitors may be reluctant to be too involved in case finding, diagnosis and planning. If this occurs, families are left feeling unsupported and floundering as they try to organize services by themselves.

Registers

Some primary care teams have introduced *age-sex* registers or *at-risk* registers of the people in their care who are most likely to have problems. Regular visiting and proper assessment of the patients on these registers can go a long way towards foreseeing and preparing suitable care and towards helping families to see where they are going instead of having to 'wait for a crisis'.

General practitioners

Within the team the GP is not likely, if he has been qualified for many years, to have had much training about dementia and a few are still reluctant to see the importance of good co-ordination and liaison between services. There is urgent need for better education and for continuing education. Since most GPs do not have enough time to spend explaining all about dementia to families they should have access to educational literature (p. 211) to give to relatives. It should be remembered that each general practitioner is likely to have no more than 20 elderly dementing patients in their practice (a few of whom will be in care) and no more than one or two younger dementing people. Indeed, the figures may be even lower than these (see p. 65).

Health visitors

The health visitor is uniquely placed to find cases of dementia, assist in diagnosis by getting background information, plan services and support families. At best the health visitor can be a 'key worker' (p. 215), a contact point for relatives and other professionals. Sadly, despite an increasing move towards working with elderly people, many health visitors still see their core job as being with young children and their families. A vigorous campaign of retraining and persuasion is needed to help health visitors fulfil a potentially very useful role.

Community psychiatric nurses (CPN)

This specially trained nurse, if attached to a health centre, can take a more active role than the health visitor. As well as case finding she can be involved in identifying the specific problems of dementing patients and offering advice on mangement. CPNs also give specialist advice and support to relatives and link specifically with the hospital psychiatric team in planning care in the community or easing the path of the patient to day hospital or admission.

Nursing services

The district nurse or practice nurse is likely to be involved with specific nursing tasks, such as dealing with incontinence, dressings, supervision of medicines or injections. They may be involved with bathing, or there may be specific *bathing aides*, and they may offer a *'tucking in'* service or, for the severely ill patient, a *night nursing* service.

The local social work department

Home help

Out of all helping agencies the home care department gives the most valuable help to patients who live at home. Home helps have long included in their 'core' jobs a number of tasks that can help the dementing person, help with shopping, care of the house, cooking, dressing, some laundry. In the past, however, their main job has been with physically disabled people, so social supervision, social stimulation, reminiscence and recreation with dementing people have been seen as marginal interests. Now, more and more home helps are being trained and given responsibilities for dementing people and their problems. Also in many parts of the country it is being recognized that regular help only in the mornings is insufficient for many patients. A much more flexible home help service is required, offering evening visits or weekend cover, and with the ability to increase cover suddenly in an emergency, if the patient is ill or a relative goes away. Special 'augmented care' schemes with a nursing contribution as well as the home help service could go a long way towards coping with some of the crises of dementia (Table 1.4).

Social workers

The social worker is likely to become involved over specific problems. There are as yet no statutory duties of social workers concerning the care of the elderly (apart from the requirement that social work departments should provide residential care). The core of their job consists of problems of finance relating to housing, DHSS payments, family problems including complaints of poor care or violence and the organization, and planning of care in the community or in residential homes. A statutory duty to assess the needs of the disabled and their relatives has been proposed. This would create a clearer core to social workers' roles with the elderly.

There is anyway a growing trend of specialization within social work departments, and workers with a special interest in the elderly are more likely to develop a clear 'core' job and gain more satisfaction.

Specialized, approved social workers or mental health officers already have a specific job in relation to the arrangements for compulsory guardianship or hospital admission under the Mental Health Act. Any developments of 'advocacy' (p. 246) for the dementing would create a further specific role.

Unfortunately, the subject of dementia is absent or underplayed in many social work training courses. This is a gap which needs to be filled urgently. There is also a need for already trained social workers to gain more knowledge and understanding of dementia through in-service training.

Occupational therapists

The community OT is mainly concerned with the assessment of the 'activities of daily living', including dressing, washing, bathing, toileting, as well as recreational activities, and with the provision of suitable aids and adaptations. Occupational therapists need training with regard to dementia, for they must assess the patient's mental state as well as her physical deficits in order to know whether she will be able to make proper use of any aids.

Voluntary services

The title 'voluntary body' covers a vast range of different types of service. Some are small local organizations running one specific service, some are nationwide bodies offering a wide range of services, others lie between these extremes. Some are involved with the care of patients, others with the support of relatives, others act as pressure groups. Some are partially funded by the health or social services, some are completely self-financing. Some run in parallel, offering identical types of service to those offered by health or social services, some offer completely different or innovative services.

Filling gaps. For dementia sufferers and their families the voluntary bodies come into their own when they fill the gaps left by the public services, either a gap of quantity in a service or the complete absence of a particular sort of service. Voluntary groups, being less stuck in a world of cash limits and the bureaucratic delays of large organizations, can often bring new ideas into practice quicker. Thus many of the gaps in community care, such as in transport services, sitting services, night cover, small day centres for dementia sufferers, counselling services, relatives' support groups and public education have all been filled locally by the initiative of voluntary bodies.

Finance. Most of these projects need considerable sums of money, because a paid organizer and payments for staff are needed to keep them going, and to pay for premises. This, unfortunately, means that organizations have to spend much of their effort on fund raising, be it from street collections, charitable trusts, local social work or health service funds, government agencies or industry.

Continuity of support. The greatest problem for small voluntary community care projects is to keep up the impetus, especially if volunteer helpers are being used. Support, training and even supervision by established social work or health service teams, or individual professionals, can help considerably as long as it is not seen as interference — above all, voluntary bodies value and need their independence.

Meals on wheels

This service is of great importance for mildly demented people whose time sense is faulty and who are in danger of neglecting themselves. A little extra supervision is required, however, since all too often the meal is forgotten about, stored in a cupboard, thrown away, or given to the cat by dementing patients.

Transport services

Transport services are vital in the care of dementia, because of the patient's lack of motivation, poor geographical sense and poor time sense. Voluntary transport to outpatient clinics, to day care centres or for visiting contributes towards helping dementing people keep in touch with the outside world.

Sitting services

Here a volunteer stays with the patient for a few hours to offer stimulation, companionship and activity and to allow relatives a break for shopping or recreation. The sitter gives supervision, but not a home help service. Sitting services can also provide useful stimulation and orientation for dementing people who live alone. *Night sitting* can be very helpful if the patient tends to be restless, though, as in day sitting, the presence of a stranger in the house can occasionally be disturbing. *Tucking-in* refers to a visit to the patient during the evening to ensure that she goes to bed safely and at the proper time.

Day centres

The small local day centre for the dementing patient is an ideal project for a voluntary organization. Six to ten patients attend per day, and a few volunteers with one paid organizer can run an effective service. Being local, the problems of transport are lessened, and patients are less reluctant to attend.

Counselling and relatives' support groups

These are usually run by branches of the national organizations, Age Concern, the Alzheimer's Disease Society, the Huntington's Chorea Society. They can be specially useful because more time can be given than most professionals can offer, because special understanding and knowledge is built up, because other relatives share experience (p. 212), and because the organizations are independent of health and social services. Voluntary organizations can thus both know and keep in good communication with the statutory services, while at the same time listening to complaints or disappointments about services and giving advice about how to get a better deal.

Education

Information for the public through carers' guides and explanatory information on local services is invaluable to anybody trying to find their way through complicated systems of care.

Sheltered housing

The core responsibilities of sheltered housing schemes usually have little or no link with dementia. Yet inevitably there are one or two dementia sufferers in each scheme. Wardens need to know how to cope with their problems and how to educate other residents to help. Dementing people should not as a rule be segregated from 'normal' people. So the non-demented also need training and advice in how to communicate with and help their dementing neighbours, who may be forgetful, disorientated for time, wandering or distressed.

Dementia will, however, inevitably mean for some that they must leave sheltered housing. Contracts of tenancy and collaboration with social work and health services should be such that a transfer to fuller care is relatively easy. But sheltered housing schemes have to accept more dementia than is assumed in their core job.

Options

Some organizations have their own residential or nursing homes to which people can be transferred, some even on the same site (a 'geriatric campus'). Others are developing special 'care housing' for more disabled people including dementing patients. Here a small group of residents lives in a unit with individual bed/sitting rooms and communal living space supervised more closely than in ordinary sheltered housing, and with enclosed 'wandering' space in a garden or court-yard. The concept is not far from that of an 'EMI' home (p. 302), yet the patient still has her own house.

Day centres

These are usually run by the social work department or by a voluntary organization. I have already mentioned small local day centres organized especially for dementing patients. These have been developed partly because larger day centres are usually not organized to cope with dementia. The core of the large day centre's work concerns older people who wish to meet other people and engage in activities. It is assumed that they will be able to select their friends and select their activities, will take an active part in what goes on and, in most cases, make their own way to and from the centre.

Dementia. As in every other service, day centres have had to take more than their fair share of dementia sufferers, and their functions overlap with those of the day *hospitals*. As in sheltered housing there is a danger that non-demented attenders ostracize or ignore the dementing, and this is made worse if staff do not have time to break the ice, encouraging dementing members to get involved and encouraging the non-dementing to learn how to cope with forgetfulness and not be frightened by it. But although it is true that, with good supervision, a day centre can cope with a minority of mildly demented attenders, it is not possible for them to cope with a large number or with more than one or two severely demented people.

On the other hand, day *hospital* care is not necessary for patients who have been assessed and who now mainly need relief for the relative, and stimulation and activity for the patient. Thus the need for specialist day centres to cater for dementia sufferers. In country districts such specialization is not possible. A more all-embracing approach to day care is needed with the fit, the physically disabled and the mentally impaired attending together, and involving a mix of services.

Private care

Care at home

Like the voluntary sector, the private sector of care has, to some extent, grown to fill gaps left by the public services. Private help in the house, including domestic help, sitting services, nursing services and live-in help can maintain a dementing person at home for long periods. Indeed, it has been argued that providing grants to allow the less well off to buy such private care could go a long way to improve 'community care' and lessen the load on the public service institutions. However, it should be remembered that many of the helpers involved in private care are untrained and un-supervised, though proper supervision is possible in larger organizations.

Residential and nursing home care

It is in the provision of residential and nursing homes that the main growth in the private sector has occured in recent years. These homes offer an alternative to Part III or Part IV home or hospital care and can certainly alter the balance of care within an area. However, there are a number of drawbacks.

First, there is usually no co-ordination with health or social services in planning the siting and size of homes in a particular area.

Second, admission too often depends largely on the ability to pay rather than on whether the patient needs care at all, or whether this home is most suitable for her. This is attractive for those who are impatient with the lengthy assess-ment procedures of health and soial work services, and who despair of waiting lists ever moving. It exemplifies the 'balance of admission policies' idea of Table 3.6. But it can lead to misplacement. It means that sometimes the dementing person's needs and wishes are less heeded than those of the relatives. For those who can afford to pay there is little that can be done to change this. But for those who receive public money in the form of DHSS funding to go into private care, proper assessment of need and correct place-ment are necessary, and this is likely to come.

Third, standards of care have in the past not been subjected to the same scrutiny that applies to Part III and Part IV homes and to hospitals, though this also is gradually improving. Few homes are able to offer much socialization, activity, rehabili-tation or recreation. Proper supervision and training of staff are only possible in larger organizations.

Finally, the contract which should exist between staff and patient is usually made with a relative or lawyer, so there is little security for the patient and no clear agreement on what is to happen if she is no longer able to cope with living in the home.

Relation to other services

For all these reasons private care can be unsatisfactory. It can also be very good when well organized by caring staff. Looked at in relation to core and overlap, we see a very diverse set of organizations which have usually decided their core job without consulting with other services, though they are aware of the gaps. The chosen core may be quite general and vague. Some homes are 'nursing' homes, others 'residential', some accept 'confused' residents or 'psychogeriatric' cases, others do not. By setting admission criteria in isolation, the private sector can feel satisfied with the care it provides, despite occasionally falling short of what other services would consider good practice. However, it is not true that all public service care reaches good practice standards either. The public and private sectors would both be better served by good communication and joint planning so that private care can fill the real gaps in a co-ordinated manner, and without any taint of exploitation.

Local authority residential care

The core functions of residential homes are laid down in Part III of the Social Work Act (Part IV in Scotland). Thus the commonly used terms 'Part III' and 'Part IV' homes. They were set up to provide a general sort of care for people who are not too severely disabled, but they were not designed to provide specialized nursing care.

Changes of population in residential care

Several changes have forced homes away from that core responsibility. First is the increase in the very elderly population, especially of those who live alone, and those who suffer multiple handicaps. When such a person's social situation breaks down, and hospital care is not required, residential care is often the only alternative. Second, the developments of community care and sheltered housing have meant that potential mildly disabled residents are coping longer at home. Third, the scarcity of special homes for dementia and of hospital beds has ensured that a high proportion of residents in homes are dementing. In many places 60–70% of residents suffer dementia. Some homes also arrange respite admissions, and many of these short-stay residents are dementing.

This change in population takes homes far away from their original purpose. The minority, who are not dementing, have great difficulty in coping with the dementing majority, whereas they should be involved in helping them. Staff until recently have not been trained in understanding dementia. The homes have not been provided with memory aids, with enough staff for supervision, or with suitable activity programmes. And, although hospitals can exchange residents, the people they can send in return may not be much less demented than those they take away.

The core of the residential home's job has been largely destroyed. And the huge overlap with the responsibilities of hospitals or nursing homes has been unwelcome. The result is widespread dissatisfaction.

Options

There are a few options for the future. The homes could accept the change and learn to live with dementia. This is logical, but more staff would be needed and the non-dementing residents would still have problems in coping with a dementing majority. Homes could accept the greater disability of residents more easily by bringing in more nursing staff, having closer links with health services, and being more ready to exchange patients for whom they can no longer care. Or they could segregate the dementing and non-dementing, or even collect together residents from a number of homes to establish a proper home for dementia as has been done in some areas.

Many geriatric hospitals developed out of a forced change in the function of obsolete fever or tuberculosis hospitals. Perhaps a similar change will occur in the residential care system. In the meantime, the staff of homes need expert knowledge of dementia. They need to organize homes in a way that fills the gaps for dementia sufferers. They need activities that are orientating, stimulate reminiscence or retrain social behavior and encourage self-caring. And they need expert knowledge of the other health problems that dementing people may suffer.

The home for the elderly mentally infirm (EMI)

EMI homes ('continuing care homes' in Scotland) may be run by the social work department, health service, voluntary or private organizations. They are set up specifically to care for dementia sufferers, and particularly those who fall into the large gaps between the core responsibilities of sheltered housing, ordinary residential care and hospital care. The true EMI home is locally based and has day care and respite care facilities as well as providing longer term care. It allows privacy and some degree of normal lifestyle for residents, whilst offering a simple, well sign-posted environment. Its staff encourage orientation and engage the patient socially in simple and stimulating activities. The home should have a large enclosed or easily observed area for free wandering.

Advantages. Such homes avoid the difficulties of getting dementing and non-dementing people to live together. They allow specific activities to help reminiscence and reality orientation. However, a good EMI home depends crucially on having sufficient supervising staff to ensure good standards of personal care and stimulation, and on these staff maintaining enthusiasm and commitment. Staff in-service training and regular meetings with relatives who continue to be involved in the patients care can help enormously. Regular contact, supervision and exchanges from the psychogeriatric or geriatric service are essential.

General hospitals

There are many reasons why dementing patients come to the general hospital, some more related to their dementia than others. Planned operations and unconnected medical conditions are often dealt with without a great deal of trouble. But it is the problems more connected with their dementia that prove difficult to treat. Accidents in the home or outdoors, including burns and fractures, infections or constipation due to self-neglect, funny turns and small strokes in MID, superimposed acute confusional states due to minor medical illness, drug side-effects or a change in social circumstances in an already frail patient — these can all lead to the necessity of admission.

'Bed blockers'

Yet many staff in general hospitals feel that these problems are not part of their core jobs, and they dismiss the idea that being unable to cope at home because of illness brings a dementing patient within their responsibility. This sort of feeling is aggravated by the fact that in many cases the immediate cause of admission is either untreatable or else very quickly remediable, leaving a patient with dementia who is unable to go home. Furthermore, the patient may be disorientated away from her familiar surroundings (p. 54). She quickly loses touch with home and with her tasks of daily living, the unstimulating ward environment encourages withdrawal, and the family, neighbours and general practice agree that she cannot possibly manage again at home. A long wait for alternative accommodation completes the dissatisfaction of the general hospital staff, especially if the patient is disturbed in any way.

To some extent the hospitals are victims of the 'balance of admission policies' as well as the 'balance of services'. For not only do patients get admitted to general hospital because of an absence of other services, but it is also true that it is still relatively easy to get into a general hospital, compared to residential homes, geriatric or psychogeriatric hospitals with their longer assessment procedures and strict admission criteria.

Options

Once again there are a number of options for the general hospitals. They could move towards a 'geriatric' style of working using home visits, day care, more multi-disciplinary work and better liaison with the primary care team, but this would mean a big shift in their core responsibility. They could give over responsibility for some elderly patients with less acute medical problems to geriatricians, as happens in most areas. Or they could hand over responsibility for all patients over a certain age to the care of geriatricians, as happens in a few areas. Inevitably this implies a transfer of staff and beds. Whatever happens it will be impossible, like it or not, for general hospitals ever to avoid having to deal with dementing people.

The geriatric service

Geriatric services arose because some doctors saw that elderly physically ill patient very often require a different sort of medical care from that which is required by younger adults. Services which include home visiting, day care, multidisciplinary assessment, rehabilitation, attention to the social and family needs of patients and strong links with the community have developed everywhere. Inevitably, large numbers of medical geriatric patients suffer from dementia. As a 'core' responsibility, geriatric services should look after dementing patients if they also have a medical problem or need physical nursing care, but they should not have to deal with those whose main problems are behavioural and who are physically fit. Nor should they have to cope with patients who are neither very disturbed nor very physically disabled. These other groups are the responsibility of psychogeriatric services and of residential or community services respectively.

Defining clear boundaries between the different 'core' responsibilities is difficult and there are large grey areas. This does not matter so much where there is adequate provision of the various services so that tolerance is possible and transfers between the services easy. And it matters less if specialist EMI homes for dementia sufferers are available. So the balance of services is important. In areas where provision is not so good, admission policy becomes more crucial. The result is that geriatric services vary quite a lot in the number of dementing patients they deal with. But dementia remains one of the principal illnesses of geriatric medicine, and appropriate training of staff and appropriate activities in day and in-patient care are necessary.

The geriatrician. This specially trained doctor can be expected to be an expert in dementia as well as in the medical illness of old age, and much of his work overlaps with that of psychogeriatricians. A special role arises in assessing difficult medical problems in psychogeriatric patients, while in return the psychogeriatrician can assess psychiatric problems in the medical geriatric patients. This requires good 'liaison' between the two services and regular meetings to discuss problem patients. If liaison exists it can also ease transfer of patients between the two services and reduce misplacement. Liaison works best if the two services are sited in the same hospital or if, as in a few places, they have 'joint' beds.

General psychiatric services

The development of psychogeriatric services has been taken most of the burden of dementia from general psychiatric wards. Services vary, however, in deciding the responsibility for the elderly who are not dementing. Most active psychogeriatric teams see dealing with patients suffering depressions, schizophrenia or other 'functional' problems as an important part of their responsibility, but not all general psychiatrists agree with this view, especially where 'younger' old people are concerned.

Pre-senile patients. One of the worst gaps in service provision relates to dementing patients aged under 65 — the *pre-senile* group (p. 11). Most psychogeriatric services accept some responsibility for these patients but the active young person in their 40s who suffers dementia can feel and look very out of place in a psychogeriatric ward or day hospital, and the young patient with permanent brain damage after an accident, illness or operation poses slightly different problems of care (p. 42). The result is that pre-senile patients do not usually get a good deal. They do not quite fit into any form of day care, they are not very welcome in general psychiatric wards and somehow out of place in the psychogeriatric service. In addition there are not enough of them in any area to set up much of a specialized service. The support of the Alzheimer's Disease Society has been invaluable for the relatives of these patients, advising on how to obtain care and helping to organize it.

The psychogeriatric service

Although psychogeriatric services have in some places tended to lag behind geriatric services in development, it has been easier for psychiatric hospitals to separate off the elderly, or at least the elderly with dementia, into a special service. The large numbers of patients involved and the shortage of resources mean that some psychogeriatric services are still dominated by long-term care and waiting lists, but others have been able to move into a more positive way of working. The elements in a fully developed psychogeriatric service are:

1. A defined *catchment area* and *age limit*. These allow accurate assessment of the needs of the area and good liaison with community-based services.

2. *Home visits* for assessment at the request of the primary care team or social work department, carried out by the consultant or other members of the team. This allows a quick response, better assessment of family and home circumstances and better rapport with the patient and family; it allows difficult situations to be defused quickly without the need for admission that would occur if the patient had been sent directly to hospital.

3. *Outpatient facilities* for physical investigation, if possible with a medical geriatrician in attendance; and access to more sophisticated investigations.

4. A *day hospital* or hospitals placed within easy reach of all potential patients in the catchment area. The day hospital offers relief for relatives and stimulation and activity for the patients, but 'granny-sitting' should not be its sole or main function. Assessment, problem-solving, medical and psychiatric treatment, physical nursing care, rehabilitation, retraining, planning care and family support are the core functions of the day hospital. Each patient should have been assessed by members of the multi- disciplinary team and a treatment programme decided in conference. Staff can keep in good contact with relatives by going out with transport, by phone and by special meetings.

Both ambulance hours and nurses' hours of duty can unfortunately impose restrictions on the length of time day hospitals open. If we are to provide real relief for relatives when they need it, then day hospitals must have more flexible hours, including evening and weekend opening.

5. An *assessment ward*, where patients can be admitted for diagnosis if that has been difficult, for assessment and

management of particular problems, or for assessment of what type of long-term care is appropriate. *Relief admission* when a family cannot cope or the social situation has changed and regular planned *respite admissions* may also be arrranged in the assessment ward. In some wards the concept of a *'shared bed'* has been used. A number of patients take the bed for two weeks stays in rotation allowing relatives to plan breaks regularly and well in advance. The family must agree before respite admissions that they are prepared to take the patient back. If they do not agree the nature of the admission is changed and a 'respite bed' should not be used.

6. *Long-stay wards.* Patients only need to remain in psychiatric long-stay wards as long as they are restless, actively wandering, aggressive or otherwise disturbed. So there should be movement between long-stay psychogeriatric and geriatric wards, and from both to residential homes, nursing homes and family care. Long-term care should not inevitably mean care for life. It should, however, be as near as possible to the standards of normality. Stimulation, compensation for losses and the good staffing levels and practices mentioned in relation to EMI homes are important if long-stay wards are to be for more than simple basic care and containment of patients.

The psychogeriatric team

This consists of medical staff, nursing staff, social worker, occupational therapist, perhaps a physiotherapist and speech therapist, psychologist and community nurse. In relation to dementia the team has a very wide responsibility in diagnosis, assessment, management and planning care; in liaison with other services; in support of relatives; and in spreading knowledge about dementia locally. Many of these functions can be shared between members of the team, so regular team meetings and a division of labour with overlaps are essential, while each member of the team retains their 'core' responsibility.

Medical staff have prime responsibility for diagnosis, general medical care and prescription of drugs. The consultant is often in the chair at team meetings and has a major task in ensuring a fair distribution of labour within the team. The consultant may also be the first person to see the patient and directs the general course of her treatment. Junior medical staff, as well as examining patients from the psychiatric point of view, inevitably have responsibilities in the investigation and treatment of physical illness, asking help from the medical geriatrician if they are out of their depth.

Nursing staff have the day-to-day responsibility of both psychiatric and physical care for the patients, carrying out nursing procedures, be they to do with personal care, drug administration or behavioural programmes. Nurses spend most time with the patients and have a major task in observing and reporting how the patient behaves from day to day.

The social worker has a particular role in finding accommodation for patients, in dealing with housing and financial problems and in relation to the Mental Health Act. Social workers are also specially involved where family problems arise.

The *occupational therapist* assesses specific abilities in the tasks of daily living and provides advice, training and aids to patients who are at home or are going home, and to their families. OTs are also involved in the therapeutic and recreational programme of the patients as a group.

The *psychologist* is an expert in psychological testing to aid diagnosis or assess the patient's losses, and in the preparation and carrying out of behaviour modification programmes.

The *community psychiatric nurse* has the task of linking with community services, assessing and supervising patients at home and providing psychiatric nursing advice to families and other carers.

These descriptions give the bare bones of jobs within the team. Actual responsibilities are much wider, for example, helping families, liaising with community services and planning care can be carried out by all or any of the team. In some teams a key worker is delegated to take primary responsibility for a particular case. There are dangers in any team system — duplication of work, with several members carrying out an almost identical assessment; concentrating multiple efforts on an 'interesting' patient while all ignore the more routine tasks; barriers being erected between the professions out of suspicion or pride; and of the opposite, a woolly overlapping of roles with no-one getting on with their core responsibilities.

There is a further danger to which all professional groups are prone. As a profession develops its particular skills, particularly assessment skills, there is a danger that they wish to leave to others the 'dirty work' of actually carrying out management. This means that the real care of the patients is passed on either to the other professions (who resent it) or to helpers, volunteers, auxiliaries or families. Each profession needs to accept some drugery as well as what they see as their core skill.

But if these dangers are minimized teamwork is stimulating, each profession supporting the other and bringing its differing views of a particular problem together. It allows an illness like dementia with its multiple problems to be tackled comprehensively in one setting without the need for the patient or her family to be referred from one profession to another and from one place to another.

CO-ORDINATING CARE

What particularly strikes relatives when they first come across this profusion of services and professions is its complexity. Some services are in one place, others in another place, some professions work in isolation, others works in teams. What is worse, some services have to be paid for, others not. Relatives cannot be expected to know all the ins and outs of the system or systems. For that matter by no means all professionals or voluntary workers know who does what, who runs what, or how the different organizations work.

We have seen a number of different tasks that need to be carried out with the help of professionals — diagnosis, medical care, problem identification and solving, supervision, help with daily living, activity, relief for relatives, admission for care. How are families to be helped in asking for this, and in planning for the future? How are professionals to avoid unnecessary overlaps, repetition of work, gaps in care and mutual suspicion?

Education

Information on local services for dementia should be simple and readily available. The simplest way is for a local 'fact sheet' to be inserted as an appendix to one of the voluntary organization's carers' guides. Staff from the various services should be able to meet from time to time to learn how each other's services work.

Contact point

In dealing with complicated organizations it is best if the 'customers' have a particular person (or persons) whom they know they can contact, who understands what is happening, and who can communicate with all the other services involved. This key person may be the general practitioner, health visitor, community psychiatric nurse, social worker, or the staff of a day hospital or institutional care. Such a system works informally, but if it is to be made formal, all the local groups concerned must agree in conference.

Communication between services

The value of case conferences has already been discussed (p. 239). But there is a more general reason why decisions ought not to be made by one organization, or one person, in isolation. The delicate balances that exist between the services require regular contact and communication. Anyone who makes decisions or tries to run a service in isolation from the rest of the system can become suspicious of others or boast about their own service. They come to believe that others are trying to palm off unwanted patients into their service, or they believe that their service is better than others and therefore do not ask for help or advice when they need it. They may even believe both at the same time.

Seeing both the strengths and weaknesses of other services and seeing the difficulties that everybody faces in having to cope with jobs that are not in their 'core' responsibility can do much to lessen suspicion and help a more co-ordinated approach. The best communication like this occurs when organizations actually plan together and when staff train together or even exchange jobs for a while across services.

Towards a 'dementia team'

The logical extension of this better communication and decision-making is the formation of a local dementia team. At its simplest the people who make decisions in the various professions and organizations in one area can meet together to find out how each is getting on with particular patients and to make some joint decisions about what services should be offered. Referrals can be made at such a meeting and the results of referrals reported back. In this way, the psychogeriatric team, the local social work and home care teams, the primary care team and local voluntary bodies can keep an eye on problems arising in the community. Meetings may take place in the social work office, in the hospital or in the health centre. A more comprehensive approach would include those who run local residential and hospital care as well as community-based workers.

To be effective both approaches require that the catchment areas of the different services are roughly co-terminous, and sadly this is rarely the case. General practices have vague boundaries, social work department and hospital catchment area boundaries are fixed but often completely different, and much residential care has very wide or non-existent boundaries.

The concept of a dementia team could go some way towards better co-ordination of services in a local area. Such a team could be the source of information and guidance to relatives, voluntary workers and professionals; it could offer a local 'memory clinic' for those who fear or are feared to have dementia; it could from the onset plan co-ordinated care which was not a mystery to relatives; it could be the contact point for anybody worried that a dementing person was at risk of any sort (p. 227). In some areas experiments in working this way have been tried. It is unlikely that many areas will go to the extent of forming dementia teams proper, but the concepts of *dementia teamwork* could be universally applied.

In the end the care which a patient receives is a balance between what they themselves wish, what their relatives wish, the different assessments by professionals of their needs, the availability of resources, and the admission policies of the different services. It is a complicated equation, and none of the elements can be left out. Good communication is the only way to bring balanced and humane decision-making.

PLANNING SERVICES

How does a particular area ensure that it is providing services for dementia sufferers that are adequate both in range and in quantity? We know from the balance of service model that if not enough of one type of service is provided the others will suffer too much pressure. We know also that there is a changing need because of the increasing numbers of very elderly people in population, and because of demands for more and better community care coupled with a move away from care in large institutions. So there is much planning to be done.

Norms

In the past, social work departments and the health service have had responsibility to provide certain sorts of facility (mostly involving beds) and 'norms' have been laid down suggesting what is reasonable provision for a particular population. The realization that different areas differ in their demand and that the balance between services affects what is needed have rather discredited these norms, but it has proved extraordinarily difficult to define what is actually needed in any other way. It seems almost impossible to quantify exactly how many dementia sufferers there are (p. 65) and it is quite difficult to find what their problems and needs are. So there is inevitably some guesswork in planning. What we can be sure of is that few places have enough of any sort of care to allow for the continuing population explosion of very elderly people.

New developments

But it is the need for a range of services which has shifted ideas on planning most. For dementia sufferers do not only need either simple help at home or long-term care with nothing in between. The developments in the last few decades in geriatric and psychogeriatric care have largely been attempts to provide half-way houses rather than an all-or-nothing approach to care. Starting with assessment wards and day care, developments of more specialized care at home and of respite care have bridged the gap more and more. It has been difficult to decide who should provide these inter-mediate forms of care, when money is already short for providing the core responsibilities of each service. Sometimes voluntary bodies have stepped into the breach and so avoided red tape. But the gradual development of joint planning, with funding or even management shared between health, social work departments and voluntary bodies, should now allow the proper development of a more comprehensive range of care in the community. And the private sector should also be involved in this planning.

CONCLUSION

The tasks we now face are to spread knowledge of these forms of care widely, and to ensure that they are available to the huge numbers of dementia sufferers in the country. There is a long way to go before a person who develops dementia can be sure that she receives planned, co-ordinated, gradually increasing care as her dementia progresses, filling gaps as they appear, solving problems and providing for her eventual total care, and all available when she needs it. Until that happens, families will be overburdened, and services toiling to cope. When it happens we can all relax.

11

The future

The 'rising tide' of dementia in the elderly has caught the western world unawares and unprepared. As survival in the rest of the world improves and there are more and more elderly people everywhere, we can only hope against hope that the same lack of foresight does not lead to neglect and poor standards of care for millions of new dementia sufferers. In the United Kingdom we can guess how many new sufferers there will be over the coming decades, and therefore have a chance to plan adequate services. What is likely to happen?

1. The numbers of very elderly, mainly female, dementia sufferers will continue to rise. Many of these people will live alone, and have few available relatives to care. The majority will nevertheless be looked after by their families in partnership with professional and voluntary helpers.

2. The public will become more aware of the problem of dementia. They will understand the illness more and will demand an adequate range of services.

3. The statutory services will continue to lag behind the increasing need for these services, unless considerable new resources are found specifically for the care of dementia sufferers.

4. The emphasis on community care for dementia sufferers will increase. Care in large, remote institutions will decrease.

Further reading

Gilleard C 1984 Living with dementia. Croom Helm, Beckenham
Pearce J M S 1984 Dementia: a clinical approach. Blackwell, Oxford
Pitt B 1982 Psychogeriatrics, 2nd edn. Churchill Livingstone, Edinburgh
Roth M, Iversen L L (eds) 1986 Alzheimer's disease and related disorders.
  British Medical Bulletin 42 Number 1
Scottish Action on Dementia 1986 Dementia in Scotland. S A D, Edinburgh
Woods R T, Britton P G 1985 Clinical psychology with the elderly. Croom
  Helm, Beckenham

Carers' guides
Alzheimer's disease society 1984 Caring for the person with dementia.
  A D S, London
Health Education Council 1986 Who cares? H E C, London
Mace N L, Rabins P V 1985 The 36-hour day. Age Concern with Hodder and
  Stoughton, Sevenoaks

Further reading

Index